Life Matters is a powerful bool
Pastor Colin Murray. The ink in l
as he faces his own immortality.
sadness that MND can bring, bu

Colin's journey with this dis...... ......us us that God's love is the glue that holds us together and when we face life-changing and life-ending situations, whether for ourselves or Pastoral care, this book will prove invaluable.

Thank you, Colin, for sharing your journey.

Pastor Bill Jeffery, Tenerife Family Church

We all long to live together in peace and happiness, understanding and purpose. Often our lives fall into an unadventurous routine until something happens that turns our world and faith upside down.

Thoroughly shaken and standing on a shifting foundation, then does life or even faith make any sense at all?

I can recommend and believe that this book, written by Colin Murray, will help stabilise unsteady emotions, give hope, and point the reader to a helpful course of direction in their life.

Romans 5;5 – Now hope does not disappoint, because the love of God has been poured out in our hearts by the Holy Spirit who was given to us.

Rosalind Jeffrey, co-pastor of Tenerife Family Church

How do you cope when you are diagnosed with a medical condition that has no known cure and *"presents an extremely unappetising vision of the future"*?

In this book, Colin takes us on his journey, after being told he has MND, in an open and honest dialogue, opening up some of life's big questions yet keeping it all rooted and grounded in the Word, Love and Sovereignty of God.

I have witnessed at first hand the struggles, joys, and difficulties of Colin's journey and how, amidst it all, he continues to display a faith that like His Lord prays: Father, if you are willing, take this cup from me; yet not my will, but yours be done.

Graham Swanson, Pastor Elgin Baptist Church

As I read *Life Matters* from a treasured friend and brother in Christ, Colin Murray, I begin where Colin hears those devastating words from his neurologist: "Mr Murray you have Motor neurone!" This clearly took the wind right out of Colin's sails and left him in the ripple of life with the shock wave that just knocked him for six.

My immediate focus was on the Bible verse Hebrews 12:1-2 *Let us run with endurance the race that is set before us, looking to Jesus, the founder and perfecter of our faith, who for the joy that was set before him endured the cross.*

The above verse is written to encourage and challenge readers to persevere in their faith, especially in the toughest of physical trials. My dear friend Colin is a faithful man of God who knows his home is in heaven, where he is promised eternal life and to be in Glory with his Heavenly Father. His faith and fortitude shines through in this book. His endurance and determination during this trial is a remarkable testimony of his love for his Saviour.

Furthermore, his passion, commitment, and fire for Portsoy Community Church remains as high as the heavens despite his health challenges.

May God abundantly bless Colin and enlarge the tent of his ministry through this publication. May He cover His faithful servant with Angel wings and remain an ever-present fortress in these difficult times as he continues to shine brightly for Jesus.

Eddie Murison and his wife Cheryl – Evangelists
Eddie is author of *Bruised and not Broken* & *To the Extreme*

LIFE MATTERS

A Pastor Embracing Life in the Face of a Motor Neurone Diagnosis

Colin Murray

Troubador Publishing Ltd
Unit E2 Airfield Business Park
Harrison Road, Market Harborough
Leicestershire LE16 7UL
Tel: 0116 279 2299
Email: books@troubador.co.uk
Web: www.troubador.co.uk

ISBN 978-1-80514-122-8

British Library Cataloguing in Publication Data.
A catalogue record for this book is available from the British Library.

Printed and bound in the UK by TJ Books Limited, Padstow, Cornwall
Typeset in 11pt Minion Pro by Troubador Publishing Ltd, Leicester, UK

Matador is an imprint of Troubador Publishing Ltd

MIX
Paper from
responsible sources
FSC   FSC® C013056

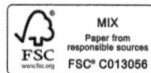

Contents

Foreword: Rev. Nigel Barton   ix
Acknowledgements   xiii

MR MURRAY, YOU HAVE MOTOR NEURONE DISEASE   1
FAITH, FORTITUDE AND POSITIVITY   3
MND – THE ORIGIN, THE MYSTERY AND
    THE MISCONCEPTIONS   6
FEAR OF DEATH   11
THE VALUE OF EMPATHY AND COMPASSION   15
SHOWING UNDERSTANDING OF SOMEONE'S
    PHYSICAL PAIN   19
UNDERSTANDING THE BREVITY OF LIFE   22
DEALING WITH REGRET   25
THE NECESSITY OF RECONCILIATION   30
WHY ME? WHY NOT ME?   34
WHO NUMBERS OUR DAYS ON EARTH?   38
HOW GOD HEALS   41
ARE MIRACLES FOR TODAY?   47
THE CRUELTY AND INSENSITIVITY OF FELLOW
    CHRISTIANS   52
MY MND INSPIRATIONS   61

MAKING SENSE OF SUFFERING   66
WHO CAUSES OUR SUFFERING?   70
A RACE OF FORTITUDE, NOT FITNESS   72
LESSONS FROM VIKTOR FRANKL   75
LEAVING A LEGACY   79
ANTICIPATORY GRIEF, STIGMA AND DENIAL   83
FEELING LOVED   86
THE COMPASSION, LOVE AND LEGACY OF
    FATHER DAMIEN   89
ONE DAY AT A TIME   92
EPILOGUE: PITY ME NOT   96

FOREWORD

REV. NIGEL BARTON

I have never had the joy and privilege of meeting Colin in the flesh, but I have been greatly encouraged and blessed, having been diagnosed with MND in 2016, by his honest, heart-warming reflections on Facebook. This spiritual instruction comes without charge which makes it even more enjoyable to a Yorkshireman renowned for being careful with his use of money!

As I write this, Colin has just marked the first anniversary of his being diagnosed with MND.

It is an indication of this very special, godly man that he endeavours to bring as much comfort and help as he can to those battling with terminal illness and those who seek to uphold and support them. Since the beginning of time itself, humankind has wrestled with the problem of suffering and death. With great perception, sensitivity and tenderness, Colin probes the acute problem of our pain: physical, mental, emotional, and spiritual, and the agonising spectre of terminal illness. The reason why the author is able to make such a valuable contribution to this critically important subject is due to the authority he has which is born from personal experience. It is very difficult to write with conviction and insight into the profound mystery of suffering unless you have walked this hard and traumatic road yourself. His illustrations of how God understands the painful struggles we are having to endure are described in a most helpful and illuminating way.

Sadly, the problem of suffering is the reason given by many people for their indifference or even antagonism to the glorious good news of the gospel. In this book the author gently confronts many of the criticisms and objections raised against biblical answers to why there is so much heartache and evil in the world. For those of a sceptical or agnostic predisposition, there should be a spiritual health warning as you may need to guard your 'faith' and understanding very carefully as a result!

For those who are just beginning to get their head around the reality of this wretched disease, Colin speaks most helpfully on the origin, mystery, and misconceptions of MND.

I love the way that he humbly speaks of the way that the Lord is using him more powerfully during this present chapter of his life and ministry, due to the fact that he is becoming more reliant on God than operating out of his own abilities and resources. He also reminds us that, for the committed believer, our earthly troubles, which last only a short time, pale in comparison to our eternal glory. Fantastic! He sensitively addresses the thorny subject of our death and concludes, 'We are rock solidly secure in God's omnipotent hands. Our life is in His hands'.

He writes with great thought and insight on the subject of empathy, and positively points out that those who face suffering or terminal illness are more likely to develop a grateful heart and deep faith than those who have not had to endure these immense struggles.

I gained much help from the way that he addresses the subject of healing. Colin gives a very positive, biblically balanced perspective on this crucially important but complex issue. As well as continually looking to the Lord for healing, we also need

a complimentary theology of suffering. The author does not mince his words when stating that the notion that God wants to heal everyone is 'a cruel and sickening myth'. Unfortunately, this misguided teaching causes a great deal of unnecessary anxiety and spiritual confusion to many people.

In a world abounding with fake news and false hope, it is so good to be able to read a book which is a genuine, true story. It is not remote and unattainable; it is a true story of Colin's encounter with a terminal illness. It helps us understand more about the complexities of MND. It encourages those who are contending with serious illnesses to persevere, give thanks for the countless blessings of daily living and be determined to remain trusting and faithful to our loving Lord no matter how great the challenges of life we may encounter. I whole heartedly recommend this book to all who are battling with terminal illness, and those unsung heroes who are alongside them, to give much needed care, comfort, and support.

ACKNOWLEDGEMENTS

This book is very much dedicated to my close family and friends who continue to care and support me through the daily battles of my MND journey. There has undoubtedly been a Divine hand involved in how certain people have come into my life, and back into my life, in my greatest hour of need. Many of them have run, swum, cycled, baked, sold items, and competed in gruelling races fundraising for MND Scotland. Their commitment to support me and in finding a cure for MND is truly humbling.

Paulina Honig, my friend of many years, through three book proofreads, as well as hundreds of articles spanning fourteen years, has been invaluable once again in the selfless proofreading, editing and formatting of this book.

I would like to sincerely thank Reverend Nigel Barton for taking the time to pen such a beautifully worded, gracious, and encouraging foreword. As a fellow MND sufferer and Church pastor I could not have asked for anyone more qualified and knowledgeable to write my book foreword. Nigel and I have never met face to face, but we are kindred spirits walking different paths while daily facing the same physical, emotional, and spiritual challenges with the wonderful promise of eternity in the distance.

I would also like to express my sincere gratitude to the diverse and talented team at Troubador Publishing for their sensitivity, professionalism and trust in me, by seeing the publication of this book through to a speedy conclusion. They were aware of the sense of urgency.

Mr Murray, You Have Motor Neurone Disease

The date was the 18th of March 2022, and I was sitting in the hospital café at Foresterhill Hospital in Aberdeen for the fourth time in just over two weeks. I glanced up at the clock on the wall and noticed I still had 45 minutes to go before my appointment with Dr Mcleod in the Neurology department. I was calm but slightly tense as I ate my customary bacon roll and sipped my mug of tea.

What I had hoped to be simply a muscle or nerve problem in my leg and a bit of arthritis or a carpal tunnel in my hand would turn out to be a bit more serious.

My clear discernment was that this appointment would be the medical conclusion from the culmination of blood tests, tests to measure the electrical activity in my muscles and nerves, as well as an MRI scan.

My memory flashed back to several incidents in the previous 12 months with two falls that had me taken by ambulance to A &E in both Aberdeen and Inverness. Six weeks of physiotherapy on my left leg and foot was to no avail. Then more symptoms occurred; a worsening and more obvious dragging of my left leg, which was affecting my balance.

I considered the worst scenario – MS or Parkinson's. I knew they were harrowing and debilitating neurological conditions, but I was also aware that advances in medical treatments meant that anyone diagnosed with either of those conditions could hope for a more prolonged life expectancy.

I made my way upstairs to the neurology department where I met Dr McLeod. I was asked to sit directly opposite where she calmly told me I had Motor Neurone Disease. I felt an instant numbness, possibly a surrealness, as I tried to take in the sheer magnitude of her words.

"Have you heard of Motor Neurone," she asked gently? "Yes," I answered, with my heart pounding and my head in a spin. As an avid football fan, I had first heard of MND more than 30 years ago when Don Revie, the former Leeds and England manager, passed away aged just 61, his body ravaged by the condition. Years later I had been aware that Jimmy Johnstone, the famous Celtic winger, had succumbed to the brutal condition around the same age. More recently, I watched from afar the devastating effect it had on both Fernando Rickson and Doddie Weir before it took their lives too.

I instantly knew that medically I was on death row but spiritually I needed to trust God more than ever before. Through a surreal daze, a Scripture flashed through my mind: "Peace I leave with you; my peace I give to you. Not as the world gives do I give to you. Let not your hearts be troubled, neither let them be afraid" (John 14:27) and at least for a short while was engulfed with the divine peace that surpasses all human understanding.

Faith, Fortitude and Positivity

For most people their MND 'journey' begins with a longish delay between the onset of symptoms and the actual diagnosis. For me, it was about a year. Like many others before me, with initial symptoms being relatively minor and with no real pain, I put off going to see my doctor for several months. The relative rarity of MND means that only few GPs have ever come across it. My GP noticed that my left leg was much thinner than my right one, so he referred me to an appropriate specialist for an MRI scan, as well as other tests. I was struggling to fasten my shirt buttons and I had to ask a neighbour for help with that on several occasions.

Within a couple of weeks of my diagnosis, I completed the decorating jobs I had started and retired from almost 43 years of full time working. During the previous 12 months, I had felt incredibly tired but had just put it down to age. Tins of paint that I could open in seconds were taking me 2–3 frustrating minutes. Often, I would fall asleep in my van at lunchtime to wake up an hour later. My key fob for the van couldn't work with my weaker right thumb, so I had to switch it to my left thumb to be able to make it click.

Fast forward 12 months and physically my deterioration continues slowly but surely, despite daily prayer and the continued prayers of many. I switch between a rollator in the house and a wheelchair when I am out and about. My leg and hand function slowly worsen, and my wrists are noticeably weaker. Lifting the tea mug at breakfast time is now a two-hand job. Even the use of quite light objects, such as a fork or toothbrush, requires great concentration, resulting in an inevitable mess!

With my hands steadily deteriorating, certain personal hygiene actions are increasingly difficult to carry out too. As I type this chapter, I am waiting for my bathroom to be adapted to become a wet room with the installation of a Closomat toilet. On completing the necessary, the touch of a button flushes the toilet while simultaneously sending a strategically aimed jet of warm water to cleanse the delicate nether regions. Release of the button stops the jet and starts a gentle flow of warm, drying air. Absolutely Wonderful!

I now rely almost entirely on my lovely sister-in-law Jennifer to shower, shave and dress me. I had never met her or my niece until they came over from the Philippines to live in Scotland and it has been so commendable how they both have fitted seamlessly into life in Portsoy. Jennifer is now my official carer and I thank God every day for her natural care, compassion, and understanding.

My brother Keith has also supported me more than I could ever have imagined, coming home to Portsoy practically every weekend since my diagnosis, and for that I am truly grateful.

Every day is a challenge, a frustration, a blessing, and always an adventure. I wake up most mornings in absolutely no pain, only stiffness and the constant leg twitch, and for a second or two I forget I have been diagnosed with this wretched muscle wasting condition. Then my heart sinks with the sobering reality of facing another day with this relatively rare illness that offers no remission – never mind a medical cure. But my advice to anyone suffering from a critical or debilitating illness would be: Never allow it to define you or become part of your identity.

I have been asked on more than one occasion if I am on anti-depressants. Well, am not on anti-depressants, because I am not depressed, although l would never judge anybody who is taking antidepressants. I do get frustrated with myself and my condition and I feel tinges of sadness from time to time, but I am not depressed. I did take a mild sedative for a couple of weeks after my diagnosis, but I generally sleep well naturally.

I don't wake up in a spiritual joy bubble but do eventually get round to thanking God every morning for the precious gift of life. Often, it dawns on me that I'm having to navigate the short distance to the toilet – a task now more daunting than climbing a 30-foot ladder on a breezy day!

Although l will never stop fighting MND and praying for healing, l am daily dealing with the reality of my condition, and I have to continually assess what l can and can't do, but I'm blessed to have a natural tendency to physically push things to the limit.

My voice has become a bit croaky and faint and is no longer strong enough for public speaking so, sadly, I may well have preached my final sermon in the Church I have pastored for more than 10 years, but l am truly at peace. The responsibility and privilege of leading a local Church is something l have held highly, but never obsessively or possessively. Like many who I greatly admire in ministry, I have always been a reluctant Church pastor.

However, we at Portsoy Community Church have been honoured and blessed by the willingness of so many gifted preachers, teachers and evangelists who come in and support us, and this will continue. I still lead our Community Church, but I pray that God can raise someone, or a couple, to lead the Church going forward. And of course, Church on a Sunday evening is non-negotiable. By God's grace and provision l will always be there.

My faith helps me through my worst moments.

MND – The Origin, the Mystery and the Misconceptions

Motor Neurone Disease in 2023, without a cure – not even remission – in its natural state presents an extremely unappetising vision of the future, although increased funding has sown seeds of optimism. Media coverage tends to be quite sensationalised, especially when dealing with people arguing for euthanasia. I notice too, that journalists often focus voyeuristically on the horrors of the physical symptoms, which can make researching the illness quite a harrowing business too.

However, I am encouraged that awareness of MND is growing all the time – even reaching the storyline of one of the UK's longest running soaps. An episode of Coronation Street focused on builder Paul Foreman's growing clumsiness and what is causing it – an eerie flashback to my own situation, dropping paintbrushes and tripping too easily. At first his symptoms are blamed on a recent car accident, but doctors ruled that out and insisted Paul undergo more tests.

I commend the *Coronation Street* producers for helping

raise awareness and being willing to work alongside the MND Association researchers developing the storyline and progression of this condition, the impact it had on Paul the builder, his loved ones, and the challenges he faced as he lost his mobility, and his ability to swallow and communicate.

I was also pleased to hear that the charity's experts advised researchers, scriptwriters, and the actors involved to ensure the portrayal was as accurate as possible within the boundaries of a television drama.

Paul, played by Peter Ash, spent time with Mike Small, who like Paul worked in the building trade and was diagnosed with MND, hearing how the early symptoms had affected him physically and emotionally. He's also followed the story of Rob Burrow, the former rugby league icon who was diagnosed with MND several years ago.

Corrie is clearly not everyone's cup of tea, but it deserves credit for choosing to tackle this misunderstood and sensitive subject – for placing MND in the living rooms of 6 million viewers, to educate people and give them a greater understanding of a disease with only 5000 sufferers in the UK.

It is difficult for any sensitive or rational person to respond to a prognosis of "about a year to 18 months". It's akin to being on death row, but I have accepted my diagnosis and its prognosis, trying to keep upbeat with faith, prayer, and positivity.

People like me with a terminal illness often write that they were inspired by their diagnosis to maximise the remainder of their time left on earth and to purge themselves of oppressive or even suicidal thoughts. However, not everyone can face the future with positivity and divine hope. The thought of imminent death is one of the great carnal fears that can land us in a tailspin of anxiety and hopelessness.

Motor Neurone Disease has been described as one of the few remaining illnesses that are still largely a mystery – and yet it claims hundreds of lives in the UK each year. MND typically sees muscles waste away after a loss of nerve cells that control movement, speech and breathing. Remarkably, it seldom affects the intellectual part of the brain and leaves eyesight and hearing unscathed, adding to its brutality and callousness. As I write this, there is no effective treatment or cure yet, and more than a third of the 1,500 people diagnosed with MND each year die within 24 months.

In the United States and Canada, the term Motor Neurone Disease usually refers to the group of disorders, while Amyotrophic Lateral Sclerosis is frequently called Lou Gehrig's Disease. In the United Kingdom and Australia, the term Motor Neurone Disease is used for Amyotrophic Lateral Sclerosis. I have been diagnosed with ALS, which covers around 75% of those diagnosed with the condition.

Henry Louis Gehrig was an American professional baseball first baseman who played 17 seasons in Major League Baseball for the New York Yankees (1923–1939). Gehrig was renowned for his prowess as a hitter and for his durability, which earned him his nickname "The Iron Horse".

The illness named after him is in fact Motor Neurone Disease, or Amyotrophic Lateral Sclerosis (ALS), a rare disorder that affects between 1 and 2 people in 100 000 and for which there is no known treatment, apart from Riluzole, which has been proven to slow down the progression of MND and possibly lengthen life expectancy by 3-4 months.

In the UK, it has struck other well-known people. The actor David Niven died of ALS in 1983, and more recently Stephen Hawking, the theoretical physicist and best-selling author, is said to have died with Motor Neurone Disease after living more that 50 years with the condition. I may be wrong, but I think Hawking may have had Primary Lateral Sclerosis (PLS), which is a very rare form of MND whereby people experience serious muscle wasting but can live a normal length of life.

For more than 80 years Motor Neurone Disease has baffled

epidemiologists and physicians alike. We do not know what causes MND, although it has been linked to contact sports, high cholesterol, and dementia. Various studies have been carried out around the world and the risk of developing MND does not appear to be affected by race, diet, or lifestyle. It does not occur in epidemics, it is not infectious, and it is said not to be caused or brought on by any other disease. It seems to be more common in men than women. It does not appear to be passed on genetically either, with less than 10% of instances of it running in families. Most people experience the onset of symptoms after the age of 40 and MND is most common in people aged between 50 and 70 years, so I sit bang in the middle of that average.

Emotional lability, known as Pseudobulbar Affect (PBA) can affect some people with MND. With this symptom, we may laugh or cry at inappropriate times, which can be distressing and difficult to stop. These responses may not match how we feel. For example, bizarrely, we may laugh when sad, or cry when happy. I do find I get emotional a lot more, and I tend to cry when I am listening to worship music.

During the tests I have had for MND, a young student nurse detected slight twitching on my arms and legs, something I had been oblivious to. This twitching is now much more regular and noticeable, particularly when I am in bed. To some extent, my whole body is affected by the progression of MND, but I look forward with great anticipation to what the Lord still has in store for me in this life and in life eternal. The medical prognosis may be bleak, but the eternal promise is anything but!

I naturally reflect on what genetic, lifestyle, or environmental factors may have triggered MND in my body. My mother died of cancer in her 40s – could this be a predisposition to developing cancer? I played a lot of football in my teens and twenties and have had a few falls and clatters at my work – could this be connected? My great granny and an aunt suffered from dementia in later years – could this be a link to MND? Decorators and electricians are the two trades linked most closely to MND and it is said that being exposed to solvents could also be a factor.

But I don't obsess about the potential triggers for this horrid condition, nor do I accept MND as my identity. I didn't even see my identity as a decorator or Church pastor – my identity remains in Christ.

I firmly believe that God is using me more powerfully and potently through this illness, as I become more reliant on Him. I sense that many people, who don't claim to be 'religious' or 'churchy', have not only been watching my public battle with MND but also how I respond to it. Furthermore, I am more convinced than ever that God will keep giving me the strength to endure. Paul reminds us that our earthly troubles, which last only a short time, pale in comparison to our eternal glory. (Philippians 4:13)

I realise more than ever that Heaven is my home, although I am not saying I am homesick! And that's only because I don't really grasp the awesomeness and perfection of Heaven.

Fear of Death

According to psychiatrists, at least 60 percent of adults admit to having at least one unreasonable fear, although research to date is not clear on why these fears manifest themselves. My unreasonable fear has always been rats! And for many years I had a fear of public speaking – quite challenging for a Church pastor!

One theory is that humans have a genetic predisposition to fear things that were a threat to our ancestors, such as snakes, spiders, heights, or water. This, however, is difficult to verify, although people who have a first-degree relative with a specific phobia appear more likely to have the same one.

Others point to evidence that individuals fear certain things because of a previous traumatic experience with them, but that fails to explain the many fears without such origins. The fear of death is a more universal fear, though, but it is often because of the uncertainty of death. Are we, really, ever prepared for the inevitability of death?

Mark Twain said: "The fear of death follows from the fear of life. A man who lives fully is prepared to die at any time". This certainly offers a degree of wisdom based on the research, but I think it would be more precise to replace "lives fully" with "lives meaningfully". For some of us, perhaps, these are the same. No matter what our meaningful life looks like, start to develop it now and we'll be too busy feeling fulfilled or focused to be afraid of death.

When we have been diagnosed with a serious or terminal illness, we are probably experiencing a myriad of emotions – from intense shock and disbelief to a feeling that we're stuck in a nightmare and wishing we could wake up. And when we do wake up, we are often confronted with deep fear and uncertainty.

Denial is a common response. We may feel numb and try to continue with our daily life as if nothing has happened, or we might get angry with God, or the doctor who gave us the diagnosis, and refuse to believe it. This anger – an entirely normal response – could extend to other people, including family members, ex-partners, and friends, or the world in general.

When I was diagnosed, I was naturally stunned, yet fairly calm. Later that night, I made the mistake of going online and doing a wee bit of research into MND. Well, I stumbled across a blog where people had left comments about friends or family who had suffered from MND and one guy wrote, after losing his mum with MND, that in his view MND was a good reason to legalise euthanasia. Of course, I went to bed with that comment lodged in my brain and with feelings of hopelessness and demoralisation swirling through my mind.

I woke up in the middle of the night in a state of blind panic and for a few minutes I contemplated suicide, with the New Harbour the place to do it. But, thankfully, I dragged myself through to the kitchen for a coffee and I listened to worship music for an hour. When morning eventually dawned, I was at peace. Yes, I understood the enormity of the diagnosis, but I was also aware of the eternal promise of my God and how He would never leave me or forsake me.

People who have never believed in God or seriously considered the biblical promise of eternal life may be afraid of their own mortality and the finality of death. It is common for people to pray or to reach out to God or a higher existence when faced with the prospect of the end of their life, although if we die suddenly there is no time to make ourselves right with our Creator. As the time draws nearer, questions about life-after-death take on a sharper relevance.

When we are young and healthy, it is easy to believe in our own invincibility, and thoughts of death don't enter our minds. That's what I felt like through my teens, twenties, thirties, and forties. I never harboured any fear of death. Not that I felt invincible – at least not totally! – but I was young and healthy.

In my teens and my twenties, I was more concerned about the wellbeing of my mum and dad. My mother was diagnosed with cancer when she was 44 and sadly died years later after a brave fight. My father was both a heavy drinker and smoker and I was worried about the excesses that both were doing to his health.

Fear is an overriding emotion, and it encompasses us all to varying degrees. Those who have a faith could find a deepening of their existing belief, knowing that life doesn't end at the grave. It is often said that fear of God has no place in a Christian's life: "There is no fear in love, but perfect love casts out fear. For fear has to do with punishment, and he who fears (for himself) is not perfected in love". (1 John 4:18)

Of course, the second line of the wonderful old hymn *Amazing Grace* is not merely a once in a lifetime experience:

'Twas grace that taught my heart to fear,
And grace my fears relieved;
How precious did that grace appear,
The hour I first believed.

The truth is: In our carnality we do fear, especially when love is asleep, and we are exposed as quivering wrecks. Therefore, God has wisely ordained that these two opposite principles of love and fear should rise and fall like the two opposite scales of a balance: When one rises, the other sinks.

It is worth considering that we are not at the mercy of satan, we are not even at the mercy of Mother Nature, and we are certainly not at the mercy of man's cleverness or carelessness or evil. We are rock-solidly secure in God's omnipotent hands. Our life is in His hands.

Where else would we want that decision to lie? He is our all-wise, all-knowing, all-merciful Father in heaven, leading Jesus to say the sweetest of all words: "Do not fear those who kill the body but cannot kill the soul. Rather fear him who can destroy both soul and body in hell".

And then, ironically, after telling us to fear God, He tells us what He really means by that: "Are not two sparrows sold for a penny? And not one of them will fall to the ground apart from your Father. But even the hairs of your head are all numbered". (Picture your earthly father leaning over you, asleep in your crib, counting your hairs.) "Fear not, therefore; you are of more value than many sparrows". (Matthew 10:28–31)

The most important thing to remember regarding the inevitability of death is the truth about life. We love our family and deeply care for them – but God loves them more. We may worry about our earthly legacy – but God is more concerned with a kingdom perspective. All the plaques on the wall, all the adulation in the world won't bring the peace of mind of one simple action: Abide.

In the middle of living this life with people we love in this world, it's difficult to keep in mind that this is just a temporary condition and not a very good one at that. John reminds us: "Do not love the world nor the things in the world. If anyone loves the world, the love of the Father is not in him. For all that is in the world, the lust of the flesh and the lust of the eyes and the boastful pride of life, is not from the Father, but is from the world. The world is passing away, and also its lusts; but the one who does the will of God lives forever". (John 2:15-17)

THE VALUE OF EMPATHY
AND COMPASSION

Regardless of how distracting and entertaining our culture tries
to be, questions about the meaning of life and death somehow
edge their way into conversations in the pub, the workplace,
and at home. Times of national crisis or when world peace is
threatened bring them to the surface, as well as smaller, more
intimate moments in our own lives.

Life is unfair – often brutally unfair – and so much depends
on accidents at birth, DNA, or family background. Suffering is
not a mathematical or theological puzzle – it's a desperate human
condition. We should respond to suffering, not with judgemental
words, folded arms, or insidious looks, but with practical acts of
empathy, love, and compassion.

With the advance of MND, some people experience changes
to their thinking and behaviour, including the way they take in
information, process language, express emotion and react to
others. The effects are usually mild, but can become more severe,
so there is a great need to be surrounded by empathetic people.

What is empathy? The word was introduced in the early 1900s
as a translation for the German word "Einfühlung". Empathy is

a combination of two Greek words, "em" and "pathos", which together mean "in feeling". Empathy is our ability to recognise and share the emotions of another person. It involves, firstly, seeing someone else's situation from his or her perspective, and secondly, sharing that person's emotions including, if any, his or her distress.

Empathy is related to sympathy but is narrower in focus and is generally considered more deeply personal. Empathy is a beautiful trait to have and to share. It is something I have received in great measure during this MND journey – not from everyone who was close to me or even in Christian ministry – but from so many friends and family. It has been truly humbling.

When we are suffering, we tend to make two demands that are impossible to fulfil simultaneously: On the one hand, we want people to notice the depth of our pain and sorrow – how deeply we are in the pit of suffering, how unique and tragic our circumstances are – and on the other hand, we don't want to be made to feel that we really need the assistance of others, especially if we have enjoyed many years of good health.

In one breath, we cry out: "Help me! Can't you see I'm suffering?" In the next breath we scream: "How dare you act as though I needed you and your help?"

The sufferer doesn't want to be alone and demands not to be pitied. This makes their emotional turmoil in suffering highly combustible and unpredictable. Most of us who are seriously or terminally ill wrestle with these two opposite demands. Since we introduced the term a century ago, we've steadily taught humans to regard empathy as an improvement upon compassion or sympathy.

With compassion, we suffer with another person, while with empathy, we suffer in them – it's a total immersion into the pain, sorrow, and suffering of the afflicted.

I've found out from personal experience that those who face suffering or terminal illnesses are more likely to develop a grateful heart and deep faith than those who know only good health, material wealth and pleasure. Fertilizer may stink, but it still helps things grow.

As I was scrolling through my social media feed, I was stopped on my tracks by a post that broke my heart: A father had returned from his work to find that his teenage son had taken his own life. I was instantly filled with grief for this brother in Christ and for his family. Why did I feel such pain for a man I've never met? Even though we're not friends or family, I can relate to what he's going through because of my own experience. I can empathise with him because I lost my father that way, so I know what it feels like.

In his powerful, riveting book *Being Mortal*, Dr Atul Gawande reminds us: "People die only once". So, when facing fork-in-the-road sick and dying decisions, he writes: "They have no experience to draw on. They need doctors and nurses who are willing to have the hard discussions and say what they have seen, who will help people prepare for what is to come – and escape a warehouse oblivion that few really want".

Well, I can say that all the medical and support people of the NHS who support me, from my neurologist doctor to my local GP and from my Occupational Therapist to my MND Scotland support team are not only highly professional but also caring and compassionate.

Henri Nouwen reminds us in his wonderful book *The Wounded Healer* how our "wounds" can be a blessing in our lives and the lives of others. Our "wounds", whether grief and loss, chronic illness, or mental health conditions, provide us with the opportunity to know and understand at first hand the suffering of others. They allow us to see things that those who don't suffer similarly can't see. Woundedness from grief, rejection, betrayal, abandonment, or from physical decline, fosters empathy and understanding and binds us together in our shared, broken humanity.

And for those of us with the faith to see it, our "wound" is a means by which we can access God, but not to blame God for our suffering or loss, nor to relentlessly beg God to remove it from our lives. Rather, when we suffer, we draw close to the very character of the God-who-suffers. As we examine the "wounds" in our life, could it be that rather than revealing the absence of God in our life, they are the cracks through which the light of God can shine?

As I write this chapter, I was looking to cash in a small pension fund that was due to naturally mature when I am 74! Apparently, if my doctor can confirm l will die within a year, l won't get taxed on the money due . . . Charming!

I appreciate that all savings and pension funds require clear terms of agreement, but seriously, how heartless can we humans be? To be fair, the gentleman I spoke to was just reminding me of the terms of agreement, but nobody knows for certain what the next 24 hours will bring, never mind the next 52 weeks. As we are reminded: "Yet you do not know what your life will be like tomorrow. For you are just a vapor that appears for a little while, and then vanishes away". (James 4 v14)

l am not seeking to be bullish, but l fully expect to be alive this time next year, and well beyond.

Showing Understanding
of Someone's Physical Pain

As I enter my third year battling this wretched merciless MND, I can still sleep well enough, and I am relatively pain free. Yes, I suffer discomfort with a slowly weakening body, but my heart goes out to those of you who are struggling with physical pain, even severe physical pain.

I have occasionally heard from fellow believers that pain is a good thing, referring to leprosy and such like, because it is a sharp indication that something is wrong. Feeling pain may be necessary in certain situations but it is never 'good'. I find that such a view is more about others finding a feeble answer to the unease they feel spiritually regarding someone's pain.

How easily we tire of those who continually complain of a sore back or such like. They may look fine, no grimacing, not even hunched, and it's tempting to think they might be playing on it. Possibly they are, but probably they are not, so let us err on the side caution and treat people's ailments as real and show them genuine empathy and compassion.

I firmly believe that emotions, particularly those that are suppressed and unexpressed, have a physical effect. Unexpressed emotions tend to stay in the body like small ticking time bombs

– they are illnesses in incubation. That's why we need to keep a positive outlook on life at all times, and in all situations.

Anger is a basic human emotion that is often supressed. It releases adrenaline, which increases muscle tension and speeds up breathing. This is the "fight" part of the "fight/flight/freeze" response. It can be mobilising at times; however, if it's not adequately managed, this response can lead to long-term physical consequences, particularly heart related.

We should never minimise or over-spiritualise anyone's struggle with pain. Yes, there are hypochondriacs and those who imagine pain more than feel it, but physical pain is real and often debilitating. Praise God for secular as well as Christian support groups. Often, secular groups are more compassionate, empathetic, and Christlike than Christians with their unquestionable doctrine.

The fellowship of those who struggle daily with physical pain is massive, bound together by a gentle, loving "I know," "I care", or "I am not sure what to say", where no one makes condemning suggestions on how we should be thinking or arrogantly become the divine barometer of the strength of our faith.

Praise God for genuine friendships free of "I ought to have done" and "I should have done". Pain is not the time or place for any of us to Lord over another. May God bless you and heal you this day, be it naturally, supernaturally, or through medical science, if you are struggling with physical pain.

God heals and wants us to be pain-free, but He does not heal on tap, as I have reiterated several times in this book. The same power that raised Jesus from the dead can still heal us today. Prayer is powerful and we should never tire of praying for physical healing.

I'll always accept prayer and I hope you will too.

When we suffer physical pain without blaming or cursing God and without forsaking Christ, but declaring ourselves to be His friend and servant, His disciple, His follower, and a great lover of His glory and faithfulness, we make it plain to others that having Christ in our life is more precious to us than being free from physical pain.

Scripture directs our attention away from earth and reminds us that the months and years of physical suffering are not meaningless – they are not pointless, they are not in vain. They are moulding our character, producing a greater weight of glory in Heaven. That's more than saying to die is gain, which can sound a bit masochistic! Rather, it's reminding us that the often long, drawn-out discomfort and pain we suffer in this world is producing greater gain in eternity.

With every thrust of numbing or aching pain, we can say, if we have the faith and fortitude to do so: "God will make it up to us. He will make it up to me. It will not be in vain".

In Heaven, we will look back on all those years of harrowing aches and pains and say: "It was worth it. He has made it worth it. In the words of Apostle Paul, who had more than his share of pain and affliction: "This momentary affliction is preparing us for an eternal weight of glory beyond all comparison". (2 Corinthians 4:17)

Remarkably, the pain then becomes a suffering with Christ because we are walking with Him, we are holding fast to Him, rather than discarding or cursing Him because of our pain. I can't say whether I will remain relatively pain-free as I fight this condition every day, but I thank the Lord for every day I am not in constant physical pain.

Ultimately, God is the Great Physician. Nothing is too hard for Him. To be with Him in heaven would be my great pleasure. If that is His will, I embrace it with joyful hope. But there is work to do: There is a Church family to care for, a Church to server, souls to win, a Nation to win for Christ – and the second coming of Jesus Christ to hope for.

So, for as long as I am drawing breath, I will constantly ask to be raised up for His great glory.

Understanding the Brevity of Life

Why was it that when we were bairns our days were so long? After school, we guzzled our supper and headed straight for the playing park in Portsoy at around 5.30pm and played football until 11pm, before we made our way home cream crackered! But that is no longer the case now, as I struggle to make my way to bed each night and it feels as though it was only a few minutes ago that I was getting out of bed in the morning.

When I was a young loon, I thought there were three types of people in the world: The aged, the young adults, and the bairns. Or, to put it in my childish thought-pattern then, our grandparents, our parents and us. To my young, immature, maverick mind things were meant to remain that way for ever. Of course, reality has since caught up with me.

I am no longer making 'hutties' at Kirkies Wood or spending the whole summer at the Portsoy outdoor pool, and I am long past the age when young ladies look admiringly at me twice.

I am also at an age with a condition, where going to the gym or going for a walk out the braes is going to be a fading memory. The stubborn and undeniable fact, therefore, is that soon – and very soon – I will be dead and buried. The reality of the brevity of life is a disturbingly perplexing fact.

Mature Christians know that life brings tribulation and trouble as well as blessings and comfort. Pain and sorrow are inevitable in this life. Why then is the thought of terminal illness such a shock? Why was it such a shock to me? Is it because death is such an infrequent visitor to our planet? Is it because death only comes on the scene in swift moments of devastation, so that we are never prepared? Or is it that we prefer to avoid all talk of the notion of death and are hedging our bets? Hedging what bets, you may ask? Hedging our bets that as a 'good person' we will go to heaven. The Bible documents the fact: "All have sinned and fall short of the glory of God".

From the Biblical perspective, we can conclude that we are all afflicted with terminal illness. We are all on death row -for some of us that may be five months, for others fifty years. Yet, we deny the symptoms and refuse to face up to the brevity and precariousness of life. No wonder we are so shocked when the doctor drops the "terminal illness" bombshell.

What is that omnipresent illness whose marks are upon us all and which is so pervasive that none can escape its power? It is the disease of sin, a congenital disease inherited from our fathers, undeniably and unquestionably the cause of our grief. Life presents us with the symptoms.

The sobering inevitability of being born is that we will someday die. The threat is not imaginary for we know that we must all die one day, whether from natural causes – infection, accident, deterioration, or from some other cause. Nor is there any guarantee for any of us that we shall live the full "threescore and ten". Some of us will never complete a score, while a few of us will live to be a hundred and receive a card from King Charles.

'The Author of Life' has offered, to everyone who is willing to receive it, the gift of eternal life. So far, more than two Billion people around the world have accepted His wonderful gift. And, upon accepting that gift, God grants sufficient evidence in the present life to convince us that death or the grave will not have the final word.

Ultimately, God sent His Son to provide us with a living example of how grace, forgiveness, mercy, and love could triumph over sin, death, and eternal judgement. Jesus deliberately allowed the sin of this world to be put upon Him and experienced the cruel barbaric death by means of a Roman cross. But that was not the end. God raised Him from the dead and now He sits at the right hand of the Father and lives to die no more. In that triumphant act He took the sting from death and blazed the trail for all those who will put their faith in Him. The ultimate cure for our terminal illness lies in the hands of God. That cure is affected through faith in His Son, Jesus Christ!

When our brief, earthly life comes to an end, let us not begrudge God for not adding an extra 10 or 20 years to our short sojourn on this planet; rather, let's feel privileged that our life has counted in the many hearts we've touched and the building of God's eternal kingdom.

As we pass on the baton to the next generation, we can say in unison with Paul: "The time has come for my departure. I have fought the good fight, I have finished the race, I have kept the faith. Now there is in store for me the crown of righteousness, which the Lord, the righteous Judge, will award to me on that day". (2 Timothy 4:6-8)

Revelation describes the total and complete defeat of all sin and evil in this beautiful verse: "And God shall wipe away all tears from their eyes; and there shall be no more death, neither sorrow, nor crying, neither shall there be any more pain: for the former things are passed away". (Revelation 21 v 4)

This is the reality that comes about when God has enacted His judgment and we have placed our trust in Him. All wrongs are made right, and all pain and suffering has gone.

Dealing with Regret

In 1981, a young American man named Bruce was on a train journey through northern France when a pretty brunette called Sandra boarded at Paris and sat next to him. Conversation came easily and it was clear there was a mutual attraction, and soon they were giggling and holding hands.

When they reached her destination – a train station in rural Belgium – they passionately kissed and, on a romantic impulse Bruce considered jumping off the train with her to see where life may lead him. Instead, playing it safe, he quickly scribbled his name and his parents' address on a scrap of paper and gave it to her.

Almost as soon as the train doors had closed, Bruce regretted not having gone with his gut feeling. Soon after his return to the US, he received a letter from Sandra: "Maybe it's crazy, but when I think about you, I'm smiling," it said, but – mysteriously – contained no return address.

In the decades since that encounter, Bruce never stopped wondering what might have happened if he'd stepped down onto that platform.

I am drawn to this story, because I see snapshots of my own life that had some similarities to the young American's experience:

In 1981, I met a lovely brunette girl in Bavaria, Germany but I let potential romance slip through my fingers due to nervousness and a lack of confidence. A split-second decision can shape your life in a positive or negative way.

Most of us live with regrets. In this, the season of my life with declining physical health and being unable to work, it would be easy for me to be overwhelmed with regrets.

I could reflect upon not having cared more for my parents, not having been more mature and loving in several relationships, the mistakes I made in more than 34 years of business, and all the errors of judgement I made as a Church pastor.

A life without regrets is built on a mirage – it is a delusion. If we don't see mistakes when we're looking back over our lives, and we don't regret those mistakes, we're denying reality. We're not feeling reality. We are bordering on narcissism. We have fallen short of what was expected of us.

There will have been stinking attitudes, spiteful words, deeds that were not for the glory of God but selfish ones, not loving but uncaring, and not stemming from faith but from fear, judgement, and insecurity.

We may wish we had the courage to live a life in which we are true to ourselves, not living a life that others expected of us. We may feel this, even though we are not terminally ill. This is a common regret of most of us.

When we realise that our life may be ebbing away, we look back with deep regret and we become aware of how many dreams have gone unfulfilled. Most of us have not honoured even half the dreams we had as teenagers or young adults. We may even cringe at some of the choices we made, or choices we didn't make but should have. Health brings a freedom very few of us realise or appreciate, until we no longer have it.

Plenty of things came out of our mouths that were not designed for building people up, and plenty of seemingly righteous paths were taken with dodgy motives.

In her book, *The Cultivated Life*, author Susan S. Phillips writes about the importance of maintaining friendships, especially in old age. She shares about Australian palliative care nurse Bronnie Ware who worked with people who have chosen to die in their own homes. As they approached death, she had asked her patients whether they had regrets. Letting friendships lapse was one of the top five regrets people mentioned at the ends of their lives.

Ware writes that many of her patients had become so caught up in their own lives that they let golden relationships slip by over the years. There were many deep regrets about not giving friendships the time and effort that they deserved. Everyone misses their friends when in good health, so also when they are dying. I think we all regret the loss of a friendship, whether through misunderstanding, betrayal, or simply growing apart. Yet, our culture offers little instruction about maintaining friendships. Doing so is both a social and spiritual discipline.

My 20-year chapter as a follower of Jesus (11 as a local Church pastor) is almost complete. It had a beginning: 2003. It will have an ending in the Lord's time. And every second of it – every word spoken, every attitude felt, every mistake made, every spark of inspiration, every deed done or undone – is written in the Lamb's book of life, and it is more fixed and unchangeable than Mount Everest. Nothing I do now – absolutely nothing – can make those years better or worse, more successful, or unsuccessful. That's an awesome, if quite scary, thought. I mean, that's blatantly obvious. But it doesn't hit us until we're almost done with life, and we look back. I used to think in terms of "I'm going to make my pastoring better". Now I focus on being more gracious, more compassionate, more loving.

The reality is that my memory of my past is utterly unreliable – as is your memory of your past. If we take a trip down memory lane and try to measure the spiritual successes and failures of our past, the good versus the bad, the loving versus the unloving, the helpful versus the unhelpful, we are kidding ourselves. I could cringe or puff out my chest in equal measure.

I am relieved that my memory is utterly not up to the task – for several reasons: Firstly, I have long forgotten many things entirely. I haven't forgotten the things I am proud of, but the truth is that much has been forgotten. Paul himself said: "I did baptise also the household of Stephanas. Beyond that, I do not know whether I baptised anyone else". (1 Corinthians 1:16)

Whew! thank you! Paul didn't even remember whom he baptised, which is understandable, for he baptised so many people – many more than I have. There are umpteen things I don't remember which may have been good or may have been bad – I really don't know, I genuinely can't remember them.

Secondly, I'm clueless if I try and run a fine comb over my past and attempt to figure things out. Also, the psalmist reminds me that many of my sins were hidden from me. "Who can discern his errors? Declare me innocent from hidden faults". (Psalm 19:12)

And thirdly, my memory has never been the best and I have no doubt that I have long forgotten many things. I am absolutely convinced that if I obsess over my past, I will drown in a sea of regrets.

The Old Testament prophet Jeremiah reminds us that our heart is deceitful. It is not what we want to hear but the heart tends to recall some things as good or permissible that weren't good at all so, we'll sadly end up deceiving ourselves. "The heart is deceitful above all things, and desperately sick; who can understand it?" (Jeremiah 17:9) We can so easily fake infallibility with a legalistic spirit. That's not just my heart or your heart – that's everyone's heart.

As Paul ponders his own record of faithfulness, here's what he concludes: "I am not aware of anything against myself, but I am not thereby acquitted. It is the Lord who judges me". (1 Corinthians 4:4) In other words, even a good memory and a good record is not decisive. Christ is decisive. Therefore, we need to beware of thinking too highly of our memory, whether good or bad, loving, more appreciative, more compassionate, and more loving.

It's futile living with regret. Regret can lead us to self-destruction, but God wants to use it to lead us towards true repentance. I would spend years regretting how a relationship had ended or what I had wrongly said in a certain situation. Sometimes I was subtly reminded of my folly and the feelings of regret were brought to the surface again. Now, as I face life with MND, I live life without regrets. Yes, I have made many bad decisions, some disastrous ones too, but many were made with a pure heart, even though they backfired. And the regrets I have that didn't come from a pure heart I have repented of. So, no more self-condemnation. (Romans 8 v1)

It's important to understand that regret is not the same as repentance. Esau deeply regretted his decision to sell his birth right, but he never repented of his sin (Hebrews 12:16–17). I eventually realised that regret focuses on the action that has brought sorrow; repentance focuses on the one we have offended.

The difference between mere regret and true repentance is explained here: "Godly sorrow brings repentance that leads to salvation and leaves no regret, but worldly sorrow brings death". (2nd Corinthians 7:10)

It is worth considering that two men betrayed Jesus on the night He was crucified. Judas had worldly sorrow (regret), and his life was ended. Peter had godly sorrow (repentance), and his life was totally transformed. We have the same choices those men had. When we face regret, we can let it consume our lives, or we can lay our fault at the feet of Jesus, turn from it, and let Him restore us.

THE NECESSITY OF RECONCILIATION

Everyone reacts differently to the reality that the end of life is nearing. Perhaps our advanced years are making us a bit insecure, or our health may be failing. It can make us deeply upset, very sad, or we could be more philosophical about death. Even as someone with faith and belief in the promise of eternity, I was sadder and more philosophical in my outlook. However, nearly everyone who anticipates that they are approaching the end of their life feels a need to tie up loose ends or make amends.

This need could take the form of taking practical steps to make sure that the family we leave behind will be financially secure or looked after. We may also make plans for our own funeral or memorial service, without deliberately being ghoulish or morbid.

For some of us, however, these practical matters could take second place – or perhaps they would be of equal importance to the need to re-address unresolved conflicts in our past. We may have a strong desire to rebuild a shattered relationship, to put right a wrong done in the past or in some way make peace both with ourselves and with those estranged from us.

The hankering for reconciliation in relationships is a common yearning when we sense that life is ebbing away from us. I admit, there are one or two people I would ideally like to be reconciled with; but only if that is God's will.

My nature, now that I'm battling MND, is very much one of peace and passivity, as opposed to the intensity and constant tension I felt in the early days of Church ministry. I thank God that I am now reconciled with several people I had grown apart from, or where things had become a bit strained. However, I am not vexed about being reconciled with every person I have locked horns with, in business, ministry, and in life. Hopefully, God knows my heart is not hardened towards anyone.

In truth, there is seldom a need to discuss an incident from the past, as we would seldom agree, and it may also trigger a reaction. It is sometimes enough to say: "I would like to see you again" or simply: "I am sorry that we disagreed" to open up the route to reconciliation and a place of peace. Or it may be wise to ask God to facilitate a chance meeting with the person we would like to be reconciled with.

In the Sermon on the Mount, Jesus linked reconciliation to worship and prayer in a different way to us. If our offerings of praise and worship are going to get beyond the bedroom ceiling, if they are going to come before the Throne of Almighty God, then we must be free of un-reconciled conflicts with our brothers and sisters.

Therefore, if you are offering your gift at the altar and remember that your brother has something against you, leave your gift there in front of the altar. First go and be reconciled to your brother; then come and offer your gift. (Matthew 5:23, 24 NIV)

If we are asked to visit someone who is in declining health, who perhaps desires to make their peace with us, it's worth remembering that there is no need to apportion blame, discuss a wrong, or be burdened by guilt. The past is the past and just as the person nearing the end of life may want peace and reconciliation so we too may need the comfort of knowing that we overcame any bad feeling, and we are available and willing to offer comfort and friendship for the remaining time on earth they may have.

The grace and goodness of God are on full display in the beautiful process of reconciliation. In the words of Paul in (Colossians 1:21–22, NLT): "You were his enemies, separated from him by your evil thoughts and actions. Yet now he has reconciled you to himself through the death of Christ in his physical body. As a result, he has brought you into his own presence, and you are holy and blameless as you stand before him without a single fault".

According to Paul, we have been given a "ministry of reconciliation". "Bear with each other and forgive whatever grievances you may have one against another. Forgive as the Lord forgave you". (Colossians 3:13)

At any stage of our life, particularly if we are terminally ill, when we will be able let go of any bitterness and grant forgiveness, we can almost feel the hand of God reach deep into our hearts with copious amounts of grace and mercy. When we seek forgiveness from a brother or sister we have offended, we feel a spiritual release and a peace because our heart is no longer troubled.

According to Max Lucado, the most notorious road in the world is the Via Dolorosa 'the Way of Sorrows'. According to tradition, it's the processional route in the Old City of Jerusalem. It represents the path that Jesus took on the way to His crucifixion at Calvary. The path is marked by stations frequently used by Christians for their devotions – each one a reminder of the events of Christ's final torturous journey.

Our final journey may have its pitstops too, where we can draw breath and make amends with those we have wronged or those who have wronged us along the way. I walked this path, following in the footsteps of my Lord and Saviour as a fit, healthy, and awestruck pilgrim in 2014 during a truly unforgettable trip to the Holy Land. No one knows the exact route Jesus followed that fateful Friday. But we do know where the path began: In Heaven.

Jesus began His journey when He left His home in Heaven to search of us.

The Bible has a word for this quest: Reconciliation: "God was in Christ reconciling the world to Himself". (2 Corinthians 5:19 NKJV)

Reconciliation reverses the rebellion and rekindles the cold passion that lies within us. Reconciliation touches the shoulder and pricks the conscience of us wayward, rebellious souls, and draws us homeward. The path to the cross tells us exactly how far God will go to call us back to a place of forgiveness and reconciliation.

WHY ME? WHY NOT ME?

"Why Me?" – the natural reaction when tragedy strikes or when we receive a bombshell diagnosis.

For some of us, the same question pops up when we have a flat tyre. Or catch a cold. Or get a parking ticket – Why Me, God? But life isn't fair. We learn that lesson early in life from the playground bully or when we are betrayed, wrongly accused, or lose someone we love.

Even if we know the theological explanations, they often bring no real comfort in a hospital ward or during a funeral service. Regarding suffering, as someone pragmatic, as a seeker, I sought down-to-earth answers, not textbook theories. We naturally want to know why we have been chosen for such emotional and physical pain.

We've heard it numerous times: "Why would a God who is all-good, all-knowing, and all-powerful allow bad things to happen to good people?" We can also turn the question around: "Why would an all-good, all-knowing, and all-powerful God grant a long life to bad people, such as paedophiles and serial killers?" After all, while it's heart-breaking to watch good people suffer, it feels unjust seeing evil, remorseless people live long lives.

Some might argue that Christian belief is merely an excuse to escape the harshness of reality, but that's no more reasonable than arguing that atheism is a mere excuse to escape the harsh reality of judgement and the thought of an eternity spent without God or away from Him.

I have much to be thankful for this year. March 2023 marked two years since I first felt the symptoms of MND and the first year of my diagnosis. With some neurological conditions that would not be much to write home about, but at least one third of people who have been diagnosed don't survive the first year. However, as I reflect on several traumatic events in my life before I was a Christian, I have no doubt this would have been my initial response:

"God, why did you allow my mum to die of breast cancer? What had we done as a family to deserve this?"

And then, four years later, I may have exclaimed: "God, why did you allow my father to take his own life? Was I not a good enough son?

And as a fairly new Christian pastor: "God, why are you allowing all these people to leave our Church? – two thirds of our congregation in four months – am I fit to be a pastor?"

Since then, I have stumbled towards Christian Maturity. It has not come naturally, and I am still very much a work in progress. It's become a cliché to say that we learn our most valuable lessons in pain, not pleasure, but if we are serious about our walk with Christ, we eventually learn, while suffering pain, to keep our eyes on one thing and one thing only – the cross.

While physical pain can be overwhelming, it is not the most important thing in life – Jesus is. Experiencing financial loss can be devastating, but it is not all that matters – Jesus is. The death or loss of a loved one leaves an unbearable vacuum in our days and nights – but Jesus Christ is still there.

The book of Ecclesiastes challenges us to keep our priorities in order, to be joyful in the good times and appreciative in times of struggle: "In the day of prosperity be joyful, and in the day of adversity consider; yes, God has made the one side by side with the other, to the end that man should not find out anything after him". (Ecclesiastes 7:1)

When we ask: "Why Me?" we are not necessarily being self-centred; we are looking at life as temporal, and at our present situation as permanent. Paul of Tarsus told us where to look when we cry our "Why me?" – "One thing I do: Forgetting what is behind and straining toward what is ahead, I press on toward the goal to win the prize for which God has called me heavenward in Christ Jesus." (Philippians 3:13-14, NIV)

It is hard to keep our eyes on the promise of eternity when we are living in the reality of our present situation. But when Jesus said, "I am the way and the truth and the life", He was showing us the path through all our "Why Me?" experiences. (John 14:6, NIV)

Suffering is so unfair. It steals all our attention and tries to force us to pity ourselves. But there's something suffering cannot do: It cannot steal our Jesus Christ from us and the promise of John 3 :16.

As to the specific issue of pain and suffering, C. S. Lewis, who watched his beloved wife die of cancer, put it this way: "But pain insists upon being attended to. God whispers to us in our pleasures, speaks in our conscience, but shouts in our pains: It is his megaphone to rouse a deaf world".

God's plan is for us to return to Him, and to lead the best possible life on earth. Sometimes we need to be reminded of our purpose. Pain, whether emotional, physical, or spiritual, is a sharp, unwelcomed tool to achieve that purpose. A needle may be necessary to prevent disease or infection because it prevents far greater suffering – just when what may seem even more intolerable pain now will lead to far greater happiness later.

I have much frustration living with the ravages of MND – the mundane things I could do effortlessly just 18 months ago are now a physical impossibility. I also have sadness, with the possibility of a curtailed life that may stop me enjoying a long happy life, but I am thankful for the health I still have, as well as the good health I have enjoyed for more than half a century.

Regardless of my declining health it humbles me daily to witness God's grace and goodness. From the first day of my diagnosis, I have refused to allow myself to have a "Why me?" attitude whereby I question how God had the audacity to allow something catastrophic as MND to afflict me. Why would I wish this cruel harrowing illness on anyone else?

So, I say: "Why not me?"

Who Numbers our Days on Earth?

In my Christian journey, I have gone through periods of believing that only the devil numbered my days, and I have been taught that. I now believe that only God is the giver and taker of life, though satan has some secondary role to play, but he is limited. He's not absolute. He's not decisive. He's not final. In a sense, he's always on a lead, like an untamed dog.

For example, when Job's ten children died in one day, Job says, "The Lord gave, and the Lord has taken away; blessed be the name of the Lord". (Job 1:21) And James says, "Come now, you who say, 'Today or tomorrow we will go into such and such a town and spend a year there.' ... Instead, you ought to say, 'If the Lord wills, we will live and do this or that'". (James 4:13, 15) God decides whether we live and do this or that. This promise has filled God's people with incredible courage, fortitude, and joy throughout centuries in very dangerous and life-threatening circumstances. Why is this? Because we are immortal until our Father decides to bring us home.

I look back on all my close shaves – I almost drowned in Portsoy swimming pool when I was around 10 years old, and the tumbles and falls I have had off ladders at considerable heights, as well as the white knuckle, heart-stopping moments high up ladders outside in typical NE Scotland gusty days – but these weren't the time for me to depart this world.

Until the age of forty, I felt pretty sure I would end up in heaven because I was a good person, but the Bible never promised me that, nor does the Bible promise you that. I finally came to realise that eternal life was only one heartfelt repentant prayer away. Too good to be true? I certainly believe it to be, but for many of us true repentance doesn't come easy.

When Tim Keller, an American pastor and author announced he had been diagnosed with advanced pancreatic cancer during the 2020 lockdown, thousands across the globe pledged to pray for him when he underwent treatment. Despite a terminal prognosis, and against all odds, the 72-year-old is still alive as I write this chapter. Quoting from Psalm 90 – "Teach us to number our days, that we may gain a heart of wisdom"- Keller credits his cancer diagnosis and, more specifically his own mortality, as the catalyst for the transformation of his prayer life in recent times.

Like Tim Keller, I now pray at least twice a day for complete healing, even though my doctor and neurologist told me there is no cure for MND. God can extend my life here on earth, but He doesn't have to. When I look back over my life and recognise all the things He rescued me from, I can only thank Him with all my heart.

Think of it: In the words of the great Charles Spurgeon, we are immortal until our work is done. Mortal still, but immortal also, not mini-Gods, as some preach. I may not know you by name, but your Heavenly Father knows your name.

One of my favourite songs, *He Knows My Name*, written by Tommy Walker, describes this beautifully:

I have a Maker
He formed my heart

Before even time began
My life was in His hands
He knows my name
He knows my every thought
He sees each tear that falls
And hears me when I call

I have a Father
He calls me His own
He'll never leave me
No matter where I go
He knows your name
He knows your every thought
He sees all those tears that fall
And He'll hear you when you call

We are immortal until God's work for us is done. You and I will not die until God intends for us to die. It may not be a time of our choosing, but it is His time. This is wonderful and reassuring.

How God Heals

Having been diagnosed with a terminal illness with no known cure and being a follower of Jesus, I have valued the many genuine offers for prayer, but I must discern which prayer to accept or reject. As you would imagine, I have become more aware, even sensitive, in the area of natural, medical, and divine healing.

I firmly believe that God heals today and that there are several ways in which God heals us:

Firstly – Regenerative (Natural): God created our body to heal itself; daily it fends off potential disease, heals itself from wounds, infections, and injuries. I remember falling off my bike when I was about 7 years old and was left with a three-inch gash on my forehead. My mum took me to the Pakistani doctor, who was covering for our regular local doctor – Dr Scott. I vividly remember screaming when I saw the Asian man with the turban on his head. I think I was more frightened of the doctor, simply doing his job, than getting my forehead stitched up! The wound actually opened up again a few months later, when I split my head while on the dodgems during a family holiday in Morecambe. For several years the cut mark was visible on my forehead but faded in time.

Secondly – Re-constructively: This is through the brilliant

minds of doctors, physicians of scientific knowledge for practical purposes. God allows the scientific advancement that man has discovered to bring healing to the body – medicine, surgeries, stem cells, chemotherapy etc. Again, God deserves the credit because He created man in His image and capable of making huge advances in medical science.

As soon as I was diagnosed with MND, I made plans to go over to Belgrade, Serbia, for stem cell treatment. However, I received no real encouragement, just words of caution, from the NHS. After I had done my research, stem cell treatment was a 'no brainer'. MND not only has no medical cure but also no known treatments that can potentially offer more than an extra three months of life, at best.

I spoke at length to Dr Alexandra, a specialist in regenerative medicine, a Swiss Medica doctor, and she was incredibly honest in giving me a sobering list of best and worst scenarios. I received stem cells injected into my legs and arms from a healthy placenta and umbilical cord. I also received stem cells through a nasal spray three times a day. Has my stem cell treatment been successful? Well, I wouldn't say there has been any regeneration of weakened limbs, but for several months I experienced no twitching of my arms and legs, which would suggest an element of remission.

A few months after my stem cell treatment I was visited by an Aberdeen based ITV film crew to give my views on a potential new MND breakthrough drug *Terazosin*. In studies using zebrafish, mice and stem cell models, experts demonstrated that this drug protects against the death of motor neurons by increasing their energy production. Using *Terazosin*, which has previously been shown to be effective at increasing energy production in models of stroke and Parkinson's disease, the team wanted to determine whether this drug could also protect motor neurons from MND. I am currently taking *Terazosin* but I can't say for certain if it is effective.

Of course, every human body is unique, and treatment will

respond differently for every single person. Age can be a factor, but not always. With MND we usually witness better results and longer life expectancy for those who are diagnosed in their 20s or early 30s.

A friend shared with me that a lady in her Church had refused cancer treatment because she believed God would heal her supernaturally. Tragically, as her health continued to decline, she became angry at God and eventually died. I would never advise anyone to stop prescribed medical treatment or suggest that accepting medical treatment amounted to a lack of faith.

Thirdly – restoratively or supernaturally: Sometimes God touches us and miraculously heals us, although He is no cosmic vending machine or divine genie in a bottle. This is the method that is widely disputed because it's sometimes instantaneous, miraculous, and unexplainable and fits into various theological frameworks, although many cessationists believe that God doesn't miraculously heal today. If that were the case, then there is no point in praying for healing.

It is not that the kingdom has not fully come, and all suffering and sin is being overcome now in this age. The core of Christianity is that Christ Jesus, the Son of God, came into the world at a point in history in the past to reveal what God is like and to accomplish salvation for all who believe in Him and in the fact that He died for us and is risen again. Miracles assemble around that incredibly short window in history where we witness Jesus and His apostles perform myriad miracles.

Fourthly – emotionally: Some of the most common symptoms of emotional harm are sleeplessness, detachment, depression, anger, isolation, bitterness, frustration, and fear. Some of the most common causes are betrayal, abandonment, rejection, a lack of community, and a sense of meaninglessness in life.

Unfortunately, modern culture with its lack of personal contact is a lush breeding ground for many of these emotional destroyers. We are increasingly drawn away from community towards individualism; away from trustworthy behaviour towards selfishness; away from morals that give our lives purpose towards existentialism and post-modernism that detach us from one another and our humanity; away from healthy choices and healthy practices towards instant gratification that degrades our physical health.

How can a floundering person in the depths of despair float his way up to the surface of this cultural wave and find emotional healing?

There is no quick and easy path to emotional healing. Some will say that all we need to do is accept Jesus and we will be suddenly healed of our emotional pain. But from personal experience, I can vouch that emotional healing is no hey-presto or abracadabra job. It takes time as well as the patience, care, and empathy of those around us. However, Jesus does heal those kinds of wounds that can't be cured through surgery, medication, or a positive attitude.

Psalm 147:3 comforts us with these words: "He heals the broken hearted and binds up their wounds". And the writer of Hebrews 4:15-16 reminds us: "For we do not have a high priest who cannot sympathize with our weaknesses, but One who has been tempted in all things as we are, yet without sin. So, let us draw near with confidence to the throne of grace, so that we may receive mercy and find grace to help in time of need".

Fifthly – we have spiritual healing: According to the World Christian Encyclopaedia, approximately16 million believers walk out of the Christian Church each year and most of them do not return. Spiritual healing is a huge need in the Body of Christ. Spiritual sickness and disillusionment within the Christian Church are at an all-time high. While many Church pastors leave the ministry broken, undermined, and disillusioned because of spiritual abuse, there are also a high number of people leaving Church because of abuse from pastors and other members of the congregation.

A pastor is called to be a shepherd. Shepherds who abuse the flock can expect severe punishment when the Lord returns: "He will cut him to pieces and assign him a place with the unbelievers. From everyone who has been given much, much will be demanded; and from the one who has been entrusted with much, much more will be asked". (Luke 12:46–48) With privilege comes responsibility, and those spiritual wolves who abuse their authority will have to answer to God for the harm they have done.

I have personally felt the sharp edge of demeaning brittle narcissism at least three times in more than 10 years of leading a local Church. And in all three cases I was initially met with encouragement, plausibility and all three came across as allies in ministry. In fact, I would say with 100% sincerity that spiritual abuse at its worst is more oppressive and debilitating than any physical illness, including MND. In a spiritually abusive relationship, we can feel so wounded that we can have great difficulty in asserting boundaries without feeling false guilt. We can even end up seeking external approval, rather than internal peace. In other words, we have been convinced through control and coercion that we are unimportant.

If you've been suffering from a chronic spiritual wound and doing your best to hide it – even from God – it's time to ask for healing. Confess an unforgiveness and lay your pain at His feet. Trust the Great Physician for spiritual healing.

But can I suggest there is a final way God heals and that is – eternally.

"God has set eternity in the human heart". (Ecclesiastes 3:11) In every human soul is a God-given awareness that there is something more than this transient world. And with that awareness of eternity comes a promise of ultimate healing in heaven.

The reality is, we should all be less preoccupied with our physical condition in this world and a lot more concerned with our spiritual condition, but we tend to focus more on being healed on earth.

Imagine if we could all focus our hearts and minds on heaven where we will no longer have to deal with physical challenges.

I mentioned Revelations 21 v 4 before, but we can draw such comfort from reading these words: "And God shall wipe away all tears from their eyes; and there shall be no more death, neither sorrow, nor crying, neither shall there be any more pain: for the former things are passed away".

Are Miracles for Today?

I have always grappled with the concept of miracles. As an avid football fan, I could be tempted to suggest that Darvel knocking Aberdeen out of the Scottish Cup was a miracle or that Leicester City winning the English Premiership in 2015/16 season was a miracle. "Colin, I am praying for a miracle for you" or "Colin, you need a miracle" are two common phrases I have heard, but are miracles really for today? Now that I am living with a terminal illness, I rely more than ever on a divine miracle, but does God still miraculously heal today?

What are miracles? When we attempt to define something, we find there are always exceptions. We are interested in events in Scripture such as Moses parting the Red Sea and Jesus walking on water, turning water into wine, or raising Lazarus from the dead, which are universally recognised as miracles. Those events are unquestionably super-natural or extra-ordinary in the sense that they are not explicable in natural terms. God causes everything in His creation, but on such occasions, He acts in a highly unique manner that we call supernatural.

I remember writing a blog in which I suggested that we witness miracles every day, but I now believe I was wrong. I suggested that every day we come across the small miracles that we all take for granted – a blue sky, white clouds, green leaves, diverse landscape, beautiful scenery, calm seas, and rugged mountains, But I believe the wonders of nature are not actual miracles, but more evidence of the brilliance, beauty, and diversity of our Creator.

Benjamin Warfield, the famous 19th century professor and theologian said: "A miracle is an event in the external world produced by the immediate efficiency of God". (By 'efficiency' I would assume he means God acts directly). Similarly, Louis Berkhof wrote: "A miracle is not brought about by secondary causes that operate according to the laws of nature".

Wayne Grudem, who I greatly admire, defines a miracle as "a less common kind of God's activity in which he arouses people's awe and wonder, and bears witness to himself". While miracles do bear witness to God and do arouse awe and wonder, the challenge here is that such a subjective definition greatly broadens the category of miracle but does not remove God from the event.

So that would indicate to me that someone who is born blind and is able to see in their 30s due to the advances in medical science is not the recipient of a divine miracle, although I wouldn't agree that God's hand was not on the wonder of the gaining of sight. We would be dishonouring God's power and work among us if we were to categorically dismiss the possibility of miraculous healing based on our finite awareness.

Physical healing is always a gift of God's grace, whether Supernatural or otherwise. It is clear to me that God endows some individuals with the spiritual gift of healing, but healing remains an act of God's sovereign goodness and mercy working through that individual. (1 Corinthians 12:9)

When we read about a pregnant woman, who seemed certain to be killed by a felled tree that lands on the roof of her car but misses the impact by several centimetres, we cry: "It's a miracle". When a raging fire ravages through a house as the result of an electrical fault and a family of six survives against the odds, we praise God for the miracle.

Of course, it is right to thank God in such circumstances, and we claim these incredible close shaves as miracles with the right heart and in good faith, although they may technically be wonderful escapes where God is still at work. Another wonderful story I am aware of is of a woman, blind for 12 years, instantly healed during prayer – a fully documented case now written up in a medical journal.

G. K. Chesterton made this observation about the book of Job. He said: The first part of Job is Job saying, 'I don't understand!' and the last part of Job, when God speaks, is God saying, 'You don't understand!' And there are some things that we can't reconcile. Of course, miracles do happen. I believe that. But they're miracles. They're not casual everyday occurrences.

Alan Thomas, Professor and Consultant in Psychiatry, Elder at Newcastle Reformed Evangelical Church, wrote this: "A woman diagnosed with Multiple Sclerosis is pronounced cured by her neurologist. Her Church had been praying for her and now they praise God for this miracle. A man is operated on to remove his bowel cancer but is found to have no cancer at all and his Church thanks God for answered prayer by miraculously removing his cancer. An 84-year-old celebrates that he has beaten Alzheimer's disease by living with it for 20 years. These are examples I have encountered. And the problem is that none of these people ever had these illnesses. Doctors make mistakes. They gave a wrong diagnosis. Every time a Christian declares such 'healings' to be miracles they give onlookers the impression these are same kind of healings as in the Bible. Doctors and others go away convinced that the miracles of Jesus were like these: diagnostic errors born of ignorance".

There may be much truth in this statement, but I can't believe that every reported healing is the result of a wrong diagnosis. There would be no point in praying for God's healing if that were the case. As a continuationist, I can't believe that the same God of the universe who facilitated such miracles as the Virgin birth, the ascension, and the resurrection, would be unable or unwilling to allow miracles today through the power of His spirit.

Professor Thomas goes on to explain: "Not all contemporary 'healings' are due to misdiagnosis. There are other natural explanations, such as spontaneous remission and the impact of our mind on our physical bodies. Psychological explanations often suffice to explain healings of bent backs and chronic pain".

But Mr Thomas appears to be suggesting that we can only be healed outside of a misdiagnosis if it has a medical or a psychological explanation. I tend to believe there are miraculous healings by God that have no rational explanation.

We may not always be able to clearly define the boundaries between "general" and "special" divine action, since even in special events (such as the parting of the sea in Exodus) God may use ordinary causes in extraordinary ways. (We read in Exodus that God blew back the sea with a strong wind). But plenty of events throughout history have been so extraordinary that even the most casual of observers would consider them "special" or "extraordinary". When God uses such events to draw attention to His message, we usually call them miracles. That may be technically incorrect, but God is still at work.

Faith writer Philip Yancey shares a true story of a faith healer from the United States who led a healing campaign in Cambodia where there were few Christians present. It was extremely well advertised and promoted throughout the country. At great personal cost many sick people travelled to Phnom Penh for the rally held in a soccer stadium. One of the consequences of the Vietnam war is that one in 200 Cambodians has had an amputation because of the sheer number of landmines used. Such people flocked to the crusade from all over the country.

However, despite bold promises of supernatural healing, when no amputees were healed a riot broke out in the soccer stadium. The evangelist had to be rescued by an army helicopter. Later the angry crowd besieged the evangelist's hotel forcing him to flee the country. Perhaps the evangelist had honourable motives, but how do such episodes honour the Lord Jesus? Did those attending the crusade hear the gospel and that they can be forgiven if they accept the truth of John 3:16 with the promise of eternal life because Jesus came and died for them?

I would say with totally conviction that there are three things we should always remember when we refer to the 'working of miracles':

1. Not for Self-Exaltation but for the sake of Love
2. God does not heal at will or on tap
3. The gift of healing should be pursued for the right reasons – not to promote ourselves or to impress others.

I have read stories like the 'mysterious voice' that led rescuers to find a child who survived14 hours in a submerged car. I have also heard of a woman who came back to life after having no pulse for 45 minutes. I have no reason to disbelieve these remarkable stories, and I class them as miracles, although technically they could just be remarkable examples of God at work.

We can thank God when people recover from sickness without the need to call this a miracle, but who can praise God for a miracle when someone has been completely healed of stage 4 cancer when there has been no medical misdiagnosis.

Despite the reservations of Professor Thomas and many other reformed Christians, I firmly believe miracles are very much in evidence today. There may even be fewer miracles in the Bible than we can possibly imagine, and there are probably more miracles today than I can possibly comprehend. There is a good biblical reason for why there would be a certain kind of prevalence of miracles in the Bible that is different from today.

In summing up, I believe that 'gifts of healings' and 'workings of miracles' have a place both in the Church and in the world today.

THE CRUELTY AND INSENSITIVITY OF FELLOW CHRISTIANS

There is a cruel and sickening myth that torments people who are ill, and that is the notion that God wants to heal everyone, and that if we are not healed it is always our own fault for not having enough faith, or we have unrepentant sins. Of course, as someone who enjoyed good heath for many years, I probably did not give this massive issue enough thought or even enough Biblical or historical research.

About a fortnight after I was diagnosed with MND in March, a private message appeared through social media from someone I had only met once or twice, 10-12 years ago, who told me she had lost a dear friend to MND. She went on to explain that while she was praying for her friend, she felt he needed deliverance, because MND was a neurological disease and therefore demonic. So, I was encouraged to seek deliverance – through a reliable biblical practitioner!

I have encountered the weird and whacky over the years, but I admit I was a bit taken aback about this and didn't see it coming! Following this weird logic, I wondered if God had also told her that people suffering from other neurological diseases, like MS or Parkinson's, should seek deliverance too, or even people suffering from heart disease, cancer, strokes, depression, or anxiety? While I accept all sickness is rooted in original sin, I don't accept that all illness is caused by personal sin or a lack of faith.

In researching for this book, I stumbled across the disturbing story of a young couple with a brain-damaged four-year old son who eventually died, despite fervent prayers for healing.

I was surprised, if not shocked, to read that a high-profile American evangelist and faith healer, told the grieving parents: "I don't believe this was God's will. He didn't allow this to happen. It's either my fault, your fault, both of our faults, or things that we don't understand".

According to this evangelist, the grieving couple prayed, and God showed them some areas where they had allowed fear, doubt, and unbelief in. This had hindered their faith and kept them from receiving the miracle they needed. Apparently, because they received the truth, they repented and were able to overcome that fear – implying that the parents' sin of unbelief resulted in the death of their child. Furthermore, I believe there must have been far more people than the scapegoated parents who had been praying for the child's healing.

In reading that alarming story, I would doubt that the grieving parents had a lack of faith. More like they had both faith and uncertainty, as most parents would have in such a dire situation. They were told that they were responsible and needed to repent. How cruel! How devastating and confusing for the parents who were already grieving the loss of their child.

In fact, I would go as far as to say this is blatant spiritual abuse.

Contrast this with the compassionate response of David Wilkerson in his book *Have You Ever Felt Like Giving Up Recently?* in which he tells the moving story of being at the graveside of a

5-year-old son of Christian parents, feeling perplexed about what to say by way of comfort to the devastated couple. The Lord gave him a word: "Your child has experienced the ultimate healing; he's gone home to heaven".

All this raises an enormous question: If God wants all believers to be well, why are so many believers not well, either emotionally or physically? Also, many Christians throughout history were not granted long and healthy lives, and this is still the case in recent times. Of course, we live in a fallen world with sin and sickness abound, but to tar people as sinful or lacking in faith is cruel and demoralising.

Throughout the centuries, every apostle and faith-filled servant of God has died, and many of them at an alarmingly young age. The American healing evangelist himself is getting older and his body is wasting away, just like everyone else's. We all continue to walk the path of bodily degeneration until it leads to our passing, but during this time medical science and answered prayer can prolong our lives. There is much we don't yet understand that remains a mystery. John Mellor, the Australian born healing evangelist, sadly passed away before I published this book. His death came as a shock to many, including me, because he was apparently in good health and had shown no sign of illness prior to his passing. Our hope for ultimate healing is in the resurrection and the promise of eternal life.

While God grants long lives to some of His greatest servants, like Billy Graham (age 98), Smith Wigglesworth (age 87), and Theologian J. I. Packer (age 90), many other great men and women of the faith have been taken home at a young age – George Wishart (age 33), Robert Murray McCheyne (age 29), Oswald Chambers (age 43), Dietrich Bonhoeffer (age 39), Keith Green (age 28), Jim Elliot (age 29).

William Branham, one of the pioneers of the modern-day healing revival who claimed to be a prophet with the anointing of Elijah, died at the relatively young age of 56.

Jesus told His followers: "If you abide in me, and my words abide in you, ask whatever you wish, and it will be done for you". (John 15:7) Based on this promise, it would be natural to assume that we should not be timid but rather boldly name and claim whatever we wish, and it will be done for those of us who 'ask in faith'. It's a bold and open-ended promise and, in my view, does not deal specifically with physical healing.

People who suffer want people who have suffered themselves to remind them there is hope. They are justifiably suspicious of people who appear to have lived lives of relative ease with little or no personal tragedy and who believe God heals on tap. At the pool of Bethsaida, for example, Jesus healed only one in a huge multitude (John 5) but His ministry was full of miracles, including miraculous healings. We should consider the ministry of Jesus and how few people He raised from the dead: Three. So, did He not want people to be raised from the dead? And we read again and again how many He healed, but He didn't heal all. He healed one man at the pool of Bethesda, but that didn't mean that He didn't care about those who were left paralysed.

Joni Eareckson Tada struggled with this issue for a long time. As she recounts in her book *Joni*, she sought physical healing of her quadriplegia. She prayed, and she fully believed that God would heal her.

In her words: "I certainly believed. I was calling up my girlfriends saying: Next time you see me I'm going to be running up your sidewalk. God's going to heal me".

Yet, Joni is still in a wheelchair today. More than fifty years after the accident that left her paralysed, God has still not physically healed her. God hasn't yet healed Justin Peters (Cerebral Palsy since birth) or Cannon Andrew White (MS for more than 20 years) either but continues to use them powerfully.

Someone I know very well lost her Christian mother when she was only three months old, and a previous girlfriend from a devoutly Christian family lost her sister at 15 with Leukaemia.

There are indeed things that happen in this world that we simply don't understand.

Joni's perspective is one of great faith and one that I totally agree with: God may remove our suffering, and that will be great cause for praise. But if not, He will use it. He will use anything and everything that stands in the way of His fellowship with us to glorify him. Some feel that God will never heal anyone miraculously today, but many people are healed today, and He is still the God of miracles. Others feel that God will always heal a person if he or she has enough faith. But God will not be put into either box.

The concept of divine sovereignty is often oversimplified. We tend to assume that, if God is not directly, answering our prayers in the manner that we want, then He can't be truly sovereign. Or that everything is in His will, so there is no point in praying for healing. The cartoon version of sovereignty depicts a God who must do anything that He can do, or that we want Him to do, or else He is not truly sovereign. I even get the feeling that I am a 'let down', a disappointment, to those who believe that God wants to heal everyone, because I am not yet healed. It challenges their twisted theology.

Photos of empty wheelchairs or walking sticks leaning against a wall are no true indication that anyone has been healed either. My walking stick leans against the wall in my kitchen, but that proves nothing. I do believe God can physically bring paralysed people out of chairs and heal the lame, but it shouldn't be stage-managed.

In my view, we have no iron-clad promises of health and wealth. Paul suffered his thorn in the flesh, despite his fervent and repeated prayers that it be removed. (2 Corinthians 12:7-10) Yet for all that, God has told us what to do in times of sickness. We are to call for the elders, pray for forgiveness of our sins, and have the elders anoint us with oil, as we read in James 5:14-15. God has promised to hear us and to raise us up which, in this context, surely is referring to a physical recovery rather than death and resurrection.

There is still the question why so many faithful men and women who earnestly repent still die. This 'Name and Claim' gospel is a distorted view of God by teaching that He wants to bless us with health, wealth, and happiness but cannot do so unless we have enough faith. This 'offer' is appealing to people in the Third World, most of whom live in abject poverty. But it also appeals to the wealthy West. After all, who does not want to be healthy, wealthy, and successful?

Thereby God is no longer in ultimate control – we mere mortals are. Of course, this is in complete contrast to what Scripture teaches. God does not depend upon our faith to act. Throughout Scripture and Church history we see God bless whom He chooses to bless and heal whom He chooses to heal.

Perhaps the bottom-line counsel for us should this quote by William Carey: "Expect great things from God; attempt great things for God".

And submit everything to God.

Did God not want all people to be healed? Well, of course He did. He is after all a God of love; He doesn't enjoy seeing people suffer. Yet, He didn't heal everybody and didn't raise everybody. Why? Because God's words abided in Him so that He knew this was not the time for the general resurrection from the dead. There's a certain timing for when things will happen, and it isn't always now, or when we choose.

Jesus did not come to primarily grant us health, wealth, and happiness now, although he would not withhold that from us. He came to save us from our sins so that we can have an eternity of supreme happiness with Him. Following Christ is not a ticket to all the material things men desire in this life but a ticket to eternal life. Our desire should not be to have our best life now but to have the attitude of the apostle Paul, who had learned to be content "in whatever state I am". (Philippians 4:11)

Shortly after my diagnosis, I recall watching two short You Tube videos from 2015 and 2017 of two separate people being supernaturally healed from MND through the ministry of a well-known healing evangelist. Certainly, the faith healer appeared sincere, but as someone living with MND I couldn't help asking whether these healings had been backed up medically. And in what physical condition are these people today, or are they still alive? To some people, this may come across as cynical but in the 'Health and Wealth' 'Name it and Claim it' charismatic world there are many instances of false or unsubstantiated healing claims.

I see the prosperity gospel as an idolatrous perversion of the gospel according to Jesus – simply a means to God's full blessings, primarily of health, wealth, and might, now available to those who trust and obey certain faith principles prescribed by a so called man or woman of God.

Although adherents may not agree that they pervert the gospel, we do not need a theology degree to know that prosperity theology is a great divergence from biblical truth. Jesus' primary mission here on earth was to preach good news and then bear our iniquities upon the cross.

At the heart of the Word of Faith movement is the belief in the "force of faith": It is believed that words can be used to manipulate the faith-force, and thus actually create what they believe Scripture promises (health and wealth). Laws, supposedly governing the faith-force, are said to operate independently of God's sovereign will and that God Himself is subject to these laws. This is nothing short of idolatry, distorting our faith by presenting ourselves as mini gods.

As you can imagine, people have prayed for me many times since my diagnosis, and twice I was even told that I had been healed and I just needed to claim it! Both times, I believe I received sincere prayer, but surely God would have told me first that I was healed? And yes, I may yet receive a rhema Word directly from God.

It seems Charismatic and non-charismatic Christians have different views regarding rhema and how it should be understood. Many charismatics view rhema as the voice of the Holy Spirit speaking to them now. I would personally agree with that, but the true test of the authenticity of any rhema word from God is how it compares to the whole of Scripture.

In 2018, Bill Johnson, lead Pastor of Bethel Church in America, wrote in his book *The Way of Life*: "Simply put, there is no sickness there, so there is to be none here. There is no torment or sin in Heaven, so there is to be none here. We should never again question God's will in a given situation, if in fact it involves sin, sickness, or torment. It may be challenging but it's not complicated".

No sin, sickness, and suffering – who wouldn't desire that? However, Bill Johnson failed to see that this is the reality of the new heaven and new earth and is not possible in the age in which we currently live.

However, following the loss of his wife Beni in June 2022 from cancer, a clearly bereaved Bill apportioned no blame to God and there was no reference to Beni's lack of faith for healing or unrepentant sin blocking God's healing hand as she battled the ravages of cancer. On the contrary, he humbly accepted that God is sovereign, death is still a mystery, and he acknowledges that the justifiable pain he still feels now for the loss of his beloved wife he will not feel in eternity.

He said: "God is not a vending machine that I get to put a quarter into and withdraw from Him what I want. He chooses what He gives. But it is the wicked at heart that say 'God didn't do what I wanted, He is a liar'. May I never be found critiquing God when things don't go my way".

It's my firm belief that God heals. Sometimes it's immediate, sometimes it's gradual or partial but always eventual and eternal. There is much that we do not understand that remains a mystery. God chooses to make some people physically well but, in His

Sovereign will He allows others to die in the knowledge that they will be made perfect for eternity.

There is coming a day when every crutch will be discarded, and every wheelchair melted down into medallions of redemption. And all who are suffering from MND, and all other terminal illnesses, will be doing cartwheels through the kingdom of heaven. But not yet. Not yet, we groan, waiting for the redemption of our bodies.

But the day is coming!

My MND Inspirations

I think we were all deeply saddened when we heard of the passing of Doddie Weir. I had never met him personally, but he had been synonymous with the fight against MND to raise awareness and generate the funding needed to find a medical cure. His humour, courage and positivity were contagious, even as MND relentlessly ravaged his body.

When I received the hammer blow of my own diagnosis, it didn't take me long to get drawn to the larger than life, infectious character of Doddie Weir. His relentless energy in fighting an illness without a medical cure was awe-inspiring to myself and many others, as I lapped up his interviews online during those months. He was an unrelenting campaigner and fundraiser, setting up a foundation named 'My Name'5 Doddie', which had raised £8 million for MND research by the time he died from this condition.

In March 2006, Jimmy Johnstone, the former Celtic winger, finally succumbed to the ravages of MND and died at his home in Uddingston, Lanarkshire. Wee Jinky became an active campaigner for stem cell research into MND and in 2003 recorded a charity cover of the Pogues classic song *Dirty Old Town,* with Jim Kerr of Simple Minds, to raise awareness of the condition. Billy McNeil, his captain when he played for Celtic, said following his death: "He campaigned for stem cell research knowing any cure would come too late for him just so other people could get some relief. The world has lost a fantastic man".

Wee Jimmy's wish is starting to come to fruition: In May 2022, I was able to travel to Belgrade, Serbia, with two lovely Christian friends, to receive10 days of advanced stem cell treatment.

I have never been a great rugby league fan, but I have come to really admire Rob Burrow for his relentless campaigning for all MND sufferers. In late 2022, Westminster pledged £50 million to MND researchers as part of an ongoing bid to find a cure for the condition. Burrow had previously travelled to No 10 Downing Street, with friends and family members, to campaign for increased funding.

In early March 2023, Rob Burrow was invited down to No 10 to collect a prestigious award. Burrows said: "I would like to thank the Prime Minister for this award and also the £50million commitment by his Government for MND research". In front of Prime minister Rishi Sunak, he said: "I know the first £30million is already making a huge difference and I know the remaining £20million will be available as soon as possible, as time is not a luxury that the MND community has".

And in another poignant message, he added: "I would like to accept this award on behalf of my fellow 5,000 people with MND in this country and I'd ask the Prime Minister, when he stands in the House of Commons with his fellow MPs, that he imagines six more people behind every one of those 650 MPs, each with the worst possible diagnosis in front of them.

When he does that, and makes the very important decisions his office demands, I'd ask him to do it with compassion for each of those people. Because, as my good friend Kevin Sinfield said: 'This country cares.'"

Of course, as an avid Rangers fan I was fully aware of Fernando Rickson's brave six-year fight against MND that he sadly lost in

2019. His charity raised a massive £1m in a bid to help scientists with research. Speaking to ITV news just months before he died, using eye movements to talk via a computer, Ricksen urged those in sport to do more to help to put pressure on drugs companies to find a cure. He said: "The sports world could put more pressure on the pharmaceutical companies. This disease is not lucrative enough, so it has no priority". He continued: "If tomorrow an MND epidemic came we would have a cure within a week. It's disgusting but a reality".

The former Rangers captain also opened up about his own battle with the illness: "Your body doesn't want to anymore, but your brain is functioning without problems. You start losing the ability to speak. Then the legs start to get wobbly. Then you can't lift your legs anymore and you start falling". "Don't give up" was his message to others like me, who are also inflicted with MND.

To be fair, Hearts should be highly commended for their support of MND through shirt advertising. The deal was seen as a tribute to former Hearts captain Marius Žaliūkas, who lost his fight to the disease in October 2020. Žaliūkas played more than 150 times for Hearts across six seasons before moving to Rangers. I felt a real lump in my stomach when I saw Life-long Hearts fan Stevie Morris, and fellow MND sufferer, lead the team out alongside manager Robbie Neilson before of the 2022 Scottish Cup Final at Hampden Park.

Lucy Lintott from Fochabers, situated around 16 miles west of Portsoy was diagnosed with MND in 2013, when she was only 19. Lucy always dreamed of having children but when she received the devastating news of her diagnosis, she was told she would never be able to have a family. Most people with MND don't survive beyond the first three years of diagnosis, but 10 years later, Lucy has two young children. Lucy is thought to be only the second person in the world with MND to give birth twice.

Euan MacDonald MBE was only 29 years old when he was diagnosed with MND in 2003. Following his diagnosis, Euan and his father Donald MacDonald CBE resolved to do whatever they could to ensure MND research was brought to the forefront of everyone's mind in Edinburgh and further afield.

Having both come from an investment background, they approached a group of key MND researchers at the University of Edinburgh and began discussions to establish what is now the thriving and internationally recognised centre for MND research – The Euan MacDonald Centre. He currently lives in Edinburgh with his wife and two sons and is surrounded by a supportive unit of family and friends. Beating the odds, Euan is an inspiration to many, including me!

I received the book *I choose everything* by Jozanne Moss and Reverend Michael Wenham from a dear aunt of mine and I was truly humbled and inspired by the story of two fellow MND sufferers. Jozanne, from South Africa and Michael, a Church pastor in the UK, only ever met by email. Through Jozanne's story they address the myth that pain and suffering are sent by dark powers and that God is only responsible for the good bits.

Michael explains: "We receive from God everything, both light and shade, praising Him in every circumstance, seeing all of life as His gift from beginning to end". Michael bases the book around Jozanne's story, telling it in her words and with his commentary. This allows him to address big questions such as: Why does a good God, if there is one, allow all this pain in his world?

Michael comments: "God has brought us together with the same illness and the same goal: to encourage and inspire others with the life God has purposed for us". Their story is sombre, yet wonderfully uplifting, made radiant by the faith of the two authors.

To be honest, it is perhaps unfair to pick out high profile ex-sportsmen as my MND inspirations, for there are many relatively unknown MND sufferers who face this harrowing, brutal disease with humour, courage, and positivity. I am sure they are all truly an inspiration to their family and to those around them.

Rev Nigel Barton is a wonderful man of God who has a real evangelical heart for sharing the gospel message with others. He was the minister in Shetland for several years before being diagnosed with MND, which meant him leaving the island to live in Selkirk, where he could be closer to the medical support he required. This move, however, did not end his ministry in Shetland and beyond, where he continued to show love, kindness, and pastoral concern for others.

Nigel has refused to let MND get in the way of his prayer ministry and is constantly in touch with others, offering them prayer support. He also actively encourages others in their Christian walk and likes to build people up in Christian love. During lockdown, Nigel was able to share the Gospel over ZOOM and continued to be a great example of love on a daily basis, in practical terms. Despite Nigel's deteriorating health, he continues to be both a blessing and an inspiration to all those around him.

People kindly say that I am an inspiration. I genuinely appreciate that, but I don't really feel like one, to be honest, as all I am doing is keeping on fighting the good fight. I am just dealing with a brutal health condition as best as I can. For me, the real inspirations are the many friends and family members who draw alongside me with genuine care and support. These are great human virtues that can't be faked, at least not indefinitely.

Making Sense of Suffering

It certainly can be difficult to accept some of the sorrowful and sheer shocking twists and turns that life brings our way. And there are few things that can stir the human soul more than the news of a terminal illness diagnosis. We may never understand the reasons for our trials this side of eternity, but one thing is clear: For those who love God, trials work for them, not against them. (Romans 8:28).

I do believe that God is using me more powerfully through this illness, as I become ever more reliant on Him, although this is not the path I would have chosen. Furthermore, I am more convinced than ever that God will continue to give me the strength to endure any trial, as Paul reminds me. (Philippians 4:13)

I am drawn to 1 Timothy 6:12, where Paul again urged me to fight the good fight of faith, take hold of the eternal life to which we were called. Paul reminds us that our earthly troubles, which last only a short time, pale in comparison to our eternal glory. I realise more than ever that Heaven is my home, although I am not saying that I am homesick! That is only because I don't really grasp the awesomeness and perfection of Heaven.

What we see as pain and discomfort and uncertainty our Loving sovereign Father – who ordains or allows every event during our time on earth – sees as transformation. I understand more clearly that our suffering is never meaningless. I also realise that God uses suffering to change us, soften us, to humble us, and to minister to others and, ultimately, to bring glory to His name.

Dutch priest Henri Nouwen reminds us in his wonderful book *The Wounded Healer* how our "wounds" can be a blessing in our lives and the lives of others.

Our "wounds," whether grief and loss, betrayal, chronic illness, or mental health conditions, provide us with the first-hand opportunity to know the suffering involved and empathise with the suffering of others. They allow us to see things that those who haven't experienced the level of deep suffering can't see, although we have all suffered. In its most Christlike form, empathy and understanding regarding suffering in pure heart, binds us together in our shared, broken humanity, while avoiding a pity party.

And for those of us with the faith to see it, our "wound" is a means by which we can access God – not to blame God for our suffering or loss, nor to relentlessly command God to remove it from our lives. Rather, when we suffer, we draw close to the very character of the God-who-suffers.

As we examine the "wounds" and scars in our life, could it be that rather than revealing the absence of God in our life, they are the cracks through which the light of God can shine?

C. S. Lewis, attempting to make sense of suffering in *The Problem of Pain*, says this: "We want not so much a father in heaven as a grandfather in heaven, whose plan for the universe was such that it might be said at the end of each day: 'A good time was had by all'".

I should very much like to live in a universe which was governed on such lines, but since it is abundantly clear that I don't, and since I have reason to believe nevertheless that God is love, I conclude that my conception of love needs correction.

It is common to feel lots of different emotions, including

numbness, shock, anger, sadness, and even denial, when we receive a terminal diagnosis. A question I have been asked on more than one occasion is: Are you not angry at God because you appear to have so much to live for? My simple answer is: No, why should I be? Millions of people throughout history have died with so much to live for. Suffering and terminal diagnoses bring home the truth that we are not in charge. Hearing that we have an illness that cannot be medically cured is always a massive shock, even frightening. But, whether we ourselves have a terminal diagnosis or are caring for a person who has, we don't have to go through this alone

The sensitive and often emotive issue of euthanasia naturally comes to light when we discuss people with a terminal diagnosis. All that I can say is that life is a gift from God to us all, and he should always be the ultimate giver and taker of life. I understand this better and clearer now in my position.

I have seen so many Christians embittered by the storms of life and by much less than a terminal diagnosis, but being angry at God is also essentially telling God that He has done something wrong, which He never does. I believe with all my heart that God can heal me or extend my life, but if He decides not to, I will still love Him and worship Him. And, of course, I am still alive and drawing breath and I thank God every day for that.

I came across this powerful and moving wee story on loyalty called *Quiet Servanthood* by Max Lucado, which spoke to my heart for obvious reasons:

"In the hallway of my memory hangs a photograph. It's a picture of two people – a man and a woman in the seventh decade of life. The man lies in a hospital bed in the living room, not in the hospital room. His body, for all practical purposes, is useless. Muscles have been ravaged by ALS. And even though his body is ineffective, his eyes scan the room for his partner, a woman whose age is concealed by her youthful vigour.

She willingly goes taking care of her husband. With

unswerving loyalty, she does what she's been doing for the past two years: shave him, bathe him, feed him, comb his hair, and brush his teeth. On the day we buried my father I thanked my mum for modelling the servant spirit of Christ".

Of course, Max Lucado is speaking lovingly about his own parents.

Is the follower of Jesus called to be content No Matter What? Sometimes we use such language regarding battling a terminal illness – we hear that a lot, and it's a term I have used myself. What we perhaps mean by that is the battle to keep cancer, Huntington's, MND, or any other terminal diagnosis from destroying our faith.

Whether cancer, Huntington's, or MND kills us or not is not the main issue. That's not the main battle. But believe me, it's not wrong. Don't get me wrong, it's not selfish to desperately want to be well and to fight to stay alive – that's not remotely wrong. But that's not the main fight a follower of Jesus should be fighting in desperate times. The main fight, the main race, is this: Will we keep trusting? Will we keep resting? Will we remain content in Jesus no matter what?

That's the main fight and battle – it has been for me anyway.

Who Causes Our Suffering?

When I was growing up, I hardly gave terminal illness a thought. That was until I was 20 years old when my mother was diagnosed with breast cancer. And now, more than 35 years later, diagnosed with a terminal illness, I regard it as my primary responsibility as a local Church pastor to not only nourish and strengthen faith in the love and healing power of God, but also present a balanced biblical view in divine healing. Trust me, there is no more potent weapon than the word of God for giving us an accurate plumb line when it comes to suffering and terminal illness.

If I were to give the impression that every sickness is a divine judgement on some particular sin, or that the failure to be healed instantly, or after a few days of prayer, was a clear sign of inauthentic faith, or that satan is really the ruler in this world and God is a helpless bystander while his adversary wreaks havoc on his children – then I would be greatly saddened as well as deluded.

In Romans 8:18–28. Paul reminds us: "Consider that the sufferings of this present time are not worth comparing with the glory that is to be revealed to us. For the creation waits with eager longing for the revealing of the sons of God; for the creation was subjected to futility, not of its own will but by the will of him who subjected it in hope; because the creation itself will be set free from its bondage to decay and obtain the glorious liberty of the children of God".

I would imagine the futility and corruption Paul speaks of refers to both spiritual and physical ruination. On the one hand, man in his fallen state is enslaved to his addictive nature, self-absorbed goals, foolish blunders, and prideful practice. On the other hand, there are floods, famines, volcanoes, earthquakes, tsunamis, car accidents, plane crashes, asthma, allergies, Covid, the common cold, and terminal illness, all wracking the human body with physical pain and bringing men – all men – to the dust.

Just like a coat in a warm, dark closet will get moth eaten, mouldy, and ruined, so our bodies in this fallen world are going to be ruined regardless of how we love that coat. For all creation, as Paul teaches in Romans 8 v 18-28, has been subjected to futility and enslaved to corruption while this age lasts.

Despite what prominent theologians John Piper and Tim Keller believe, our sovereign God does not smite us with illness, but He does determine who gets well, and all His decisions are for our good – even if they may be very painful and long-lasting. It was God who subjected creation to futility and corruption, and He is the one who can liberate it again We know that God is in control of all things. We also know that human choice has a meaningful impact in the world. We know that God cannot be the author of evil of any kind.

We should pray for healing, and for our strength in faith, if we remain unhealed. Sometimes, we witness healing, sometimes not. But we are always healed, either in this life or the next. The glory of God is manifested when He heals and when He gives a spirit of hope and peace to the person that He does not heal, for that, too, is grace at work.

Let's pray we might always be a people among whom God is healing, but at the same time, always allow ourselves to be full of joy, peace, and gratitude, during our sickness if we are not healed.

A Race of Fortitude, Not Fitness

The race that I and other terminally ill people are running is not a race against strong winds, torrential rain, hills, heat, or aching muscles; it's a race against the many temptations that would make us doubt God's goodness and God's love. In bed we are running. Behind rollators we are running. In a wheelchair we are running.

In such a place of vulnerability we might even doubt our families' love for us, and even our partner's, or spouse's love for us. It's a fight to stay restful and content in God through vanishing muscles or weakening bones. It's not an easy race. We may not be moving our legs or arms freely, if at all, but oh, the difficulty of this race called life! It's our Olympics, and it may have to be run flat on our back or crawling on our knees. For most of us, at the end, it will be run that way regardless of being terminally ill.

Paul reminds us in 2 Timothy 4:7, "I have fought the good fight, I have finished the race." And then he defines it: "I have kept the faith".

That is the goal for those who minister to the terminally ill, as well as those of us who are terminally ill. The focus on finishing the race and fighting the fight. And Paul makes explicit what kind of fight it is. It's the fight of keeping faith: "I kept faith. I didn't stop believing. I didn't throw in the towel of faith at the end of my life through all my troubles".

We win if we keep believing, for ultimately, it's a race against unbelief, not against time.

Since my diagnosis, I have come to realise that my house, now looking a bit run down and dated, is the dream home for someone who doesn't have a roof over their head. That kid, who constantly angers and frustrates us, is the deep longing of a couple who have been told they can't have children. The job, that does our head in with the boss who takes us for granted, is the desire of someone who is genuinely looking for employment. The partner or spouse, who often appears disorganised, disinterested, and insensitive but who is also loyal, honest, and committed is the person God has brought you together with for a reason.

That unexpected diagnosis that has left your life in turmoil can be the catalyst for reprioritising life and appreciating what's really important. Life is never perfect, but it is seldom as bad as we think it is, if we remember to count our blessings and face life with a grateful heart.

There will always be a sense of surrealness regarding my condition, as I enjoyed good health all my life, and I was working full time just over a year ago from the publication of this book. I wouldn't say I have come to terms with it – it's more a case of learning to live with it as best as I can. Rob Burrows has said he feels like a prisoner in his own body, and I can fully understand that. MND may devour physical strength, but it has no hold over mental strength and spiritual freedom.

If you have been diagnosed with a serious or terminal illness, of course pray, and believe in God's healing, but I would humbly offer this advice: Make sure that you are a true child of God, having trust in Jesus as your Saviour. It's important to retain an eternal perspective, not a terminal one. Nothing should be terminal for a follower of Jesus.

When I surrendered my life to Christ, almost twenty years ago, I felt He was going to use me, and I trust He has. But I wrongly expected to serve purely out of my strengths, not my weaknesses. It's hard to serve when you feel inadequate but, in a sense, that's when God uses us most. Every day is a challenge, a frustration, and a blessing – the mixed conundrum that reflects the ups and downs of living with MND.

So, as I mourn my physical decline and disappointments, I focus on the Christmas story and all the challenges Joseph and Mary had to overcome. My suffering is not glamorous. Neither is yours – no one's suffering is. It's messy, harrowing and humbling. And yet we can seek to glorify God in it.

The nativity highlights the way God uses our deepest pain, our humiliation, the things that we wish were different, the despised and the lowly, to bring Him the greatest glory. God's kingdom is upside down. The last shall be first, the weak shall be strong, and the foolish shall shame the wise.

No matter how dark the current chapter, all our stories can end in everlasting joy in the omnipotent Light that shone first from the little town of Bethlehem.

LESSONS FROM
VIKTOR FRANKL

More than 25 years ago, and before I became a Christian, I was fascinated by the life and philosophy of Viktor Frankl. I purchased his landmark book, *Man's Search for Meaning*, which chronicles how he survived the Holocaust at Auschwitz by finding personal meaning through the harrowing, horrific experience, which gave him the will to live through almost unfathomable abuse and human deprivation. He went on to later establish a new school of thought called logotherapy, based in the assumption that man's underlying motivator in life is to find a reason to live, even in the most unmanageable of circumstances.

I vividly recall sitting in my warm living room on a bitterly cold winter's evening, staring at a simple mug of tea with a renewed sense of appreciation after I had read a particularly harrowing piece of Frankl's book.

So, for me in this challenging season of my life it is crucially important to find purpose, focus, and a reason to live – not just survive or exist. In Scripture, we are warned about the dangers of living a life without hope or purpose: Without vision people perish. Without this vision, as Solomon writes in Proverbs 29, we inevitably give up on life and eventually drown in a sea of worthlessness and hopelessness.

As the prophet Isaiah wrote: "We hope for light, but behold, darkness, for brightness, but we walk in gloom. We grope along the wall like blind men, we grope like those who have no eyes; we stumble at midday as in the twilight, among those who are vigorous we are like dead men". (Isaiah 59:9-10)

Viktor Frankl's father, mother, brother, and wife all perished so, except for his sister, his entire family were killed in these death camps. So how could he, with practically every possession lost, suffering from hunger, cold, and brutality, with an hourly threat of death, possibly find life worth preserving?

Even in the degradation and abject misery of a concentration camp, Dr Frankl was able to exercise the most important freedom of all – the freedom to determine his own attitude and spiritual well-being. No sadistic Nazi SS guard was able to take that away from him or control the inner life of Frankl's soul. One of the ways he found the strength to fight to stay alive and not lose hope was to think of his wife. Frankl clearly saw that it was those who felt they had nothing to live for were the ones who died quickest in the concentration camp. In the same way, we live longer while facing terminal Illness if we live with a sense of purpose with joy and thankfulness in our hearts.

As he saw in the camps, those who found meaning even in the most horrendous circumstances were far more resilient to suffering than those who did not. "Everything can be taken from a man but one thing," Dr Frankl wrote, "the last of the human freedoms – to choose our attitude in any given set of circumstances." He reasoned that meaning is not only about transcending the self, but also about transcending the present moment. While happiness is an emotion felt in the present, it ultimately fades away, just as all emotions do, for all feelings of ultimate pleasure are momentary.

Dr Frankl pointed to research, indicating a strong relationship between "meaninglessness" and criminal activities, addictions, and depression. Without meaning in life, people fill the void with hedonistic pleasures, power, materialism, hatred, boredom, or neurotic obsessions and compulsions.

Viktor Frankl convinced himself that he was not a prisoner in a concentration camp but a psychotherapist taking part in an experiment. This allowed him to salvage a vestige of freedom and dignity. In a similar way, I do not view myself as a dying man or a dead man walking, but rather as someone who is being spiritually renewed and transformed on the inside, even though MND ravages my body on the outside.

Dr Frankl had found a purpose in life; to do all he could to rescue his fellow prisoners from complete despair. He did so by helping them find a reason to live. For one prisoner, it was finishing a series of travel guides. For another, it was the thought of joining a child in Canada, who needed him. My own purpose in life is to reach as many people as I can with a message of grace, mercy, and Christian love, while at the same time living life to the max with friends and family.

The wisdom that Viktor Frankl derived from his experiences in the middle of unimaginable human suffering is just as relevant now as it was then: "Being human always points and is directed to something or someone, other than oneself – be it a meaning to fulfil, or another human being to encounter. The more one forgets himself – by giving himself to a cause to serve or another person to love – the more human he is".

He tells the story of one young woman in the camp, who was about to die. She was remarkably upbeat, and she explained this unnatural cheeriness in the following way:

Until her imprisonment she had never considered spiritual matters, but in Auschwitz she had nothing accept a tiny window through which she could see the branch of a chestnut tree on which there were two blossoms. That branch seemed to speak to her: I am here – I am life, eternal life – and she was about to experience that.

Dr Frankl, reflecting on the barbarity of his fellow man and the hope of something beyond the here and now, once explained: "Our generation is realistic, for we have come to know man as he really is. After all, man is that being who invented the gas chambers of Auschwitz; however, he is also that being who has entered the gas chambers upright, with the Lord's Prayer or Shema Yisreal on his lips".

Ultimately, our faith rises and falls because we are human. It has degrees. But our eternal security does not rise and fall. It has no degrees. We must all persevere in faith, that's true, but if we are honest, there are times when our faith is the size of a mustard seed and barely visible. Yes, it is possible to be so overwhelmed with darkness that we can even question whether we really are a follower of Jesus – I understand that, but by the grace of God I remain positive and in good spirits.

Leaving a Legacy

Most people have an inner desire to make their lives count, to go beyond just existing to a place of lasting significance that outlives their time here on earth. We want our lives to mean something and make a difference. We are a society that focuses on what people do and what people have done. When we focus our time and energy on achievement and accomplishing great feats, we are not leaving a legacy – we are building a golden calf for our own Tower of Babel. Adolf Hitler left a legacy, Jimmy Saville too, both were revered, even worshipped, by millions but their legacies are reviled and tarnished beyond repair.

Ravi Zacharias was a hero of mine, and I would listen to his messages for hours and regularly quote him in my writing. Ravi Zavi's life story is heart-breaking and eye-opening. Even though the messages he preached all over the world remain relevant, inspiring, and filled with truth, his legacy is severely tarnished because of egregious sexual sin that was uncovered and rocked the evangelical world. Other prominent figures in the Christian world, like Bill Hybels, Karl Lenz, Bruxy Cavey and Mark Driscoll, also have their legacies severely damaged by their sinful conduct, although genuine repentance and restoration are available to them all.

This is a warning for us who are still living. We still have today. We still have time to repent, forsake sin, seek forgiveness and restoration where needed and build upon the foundation of our faith with things that last through the fire. So, with a sober heart and failing health, I ask myself hard questions every day.

Sir Nicholas Winton was a stockbroker in 1938 when Hitler's troops began to march into Czechoslovakia. In his gut he knew that something evil was underfoot. He quit his job and began to charter trains, raise money, and transport Jewish children out of Nazi occupied Czechoslovakia and Poland. Because of him, 699 Jewish children escaped what would have been imminent death in Nazi prison camps. Vera Gissing, one of the 699 children who escaped remarked: "He did not only save 699; he saved a generation. We have had children and grandchildren. Because of him, there are about 7,000 of us alive".

In a sense, writing this book, and others, is leaving a legacy. But a greater legacy is the impact we leave by how we treat people in the mundaneness of daily life. We can write books, even build hospitals and orphanages, and have statues erected in our name, but if our character does not match up with what can be seen with our eyes all that means nothing. In fact, without question, the most celebrated men and women in eternity will be seemingly obscure people whose names we have never heard. Many will be the unseen servants who were faithful in the humblest of circumstances.

We all want our life to make a difference, but often we don't care whether we make a lasting difference. Quite often, we just want people to like us or admire us. Or we just want to get through life as stress or conflict free as possible. However, I firmly believe we can all leave a legacy that doesn't have to be bought, owned, or attained.

What is a true legacy? It's planting seeds in our back yard we never get to see. Legacy is much more than leaving something for people. It's leaving something special in people. We can all leave a legacy of love, compassion, and integrity that dwarfs leaving material wealth or any kind of macho reputation.

We don't have to know a lot of things for our life to make a lasting difference in this world – that is why our Life Matters. The people that make a genuine difference in the world are not the people who have mastered many things, but rather those who have mastered a few important things well.

When I think of the coming generations, I am not content to only leave them a few books, blogs, and articles that celebrate the glory of God and the struggles of life. I would rather leave a legacy rooted in integrity, character, and vulnerability – even though I'd always risk falling short.

If we want our life to count, if we want the ripple effect of the pebbles we drop to become waves that reach the very ends of the earth and roll on for centuries and into eternity, we don't have to have a high IQ or even a university degree. We don't have to possess stunning looks or material wealth. We don't have to come from the perfect family or be raised in the most impressive part of town. We simply have to know a few great, majestic, unchanging Biblical truths and life principles, to be set on fire by them and live with passion and positive expectancy.

I first came across this poem, written by an anonymous author, about thirty years ago – I love it, because it speaks so powerfully and poignantly of the kind of legacy that we should all aim to leave behind:

THE MEASURE OF A MAN

Not – "How did he die?" But – "How did he live?"
Not – "What did he gain?" But – "What did he give?"
These are the units to measure the worth
Of a man as a man, regardless of birth

Not – "What was his station?" But – "Had he a heart?"
And – "How did he play his God-given part?"
Was he ever ready with a word of good cheer
To bring back a smile, to banish a tear?"

Not – "What was his church?" Nor – "What was his creed?"
But – "Had he befriended those really in need?"
Not – "What did the sketch in the newspaper say?"
But – "How many were sorry when he passed away?"

ANTICIPATORY GRIEF, STIGMA AND DENIAL

In a sense, the mourning of patients diagnosed with a terminal illness by their friends and families begins long before a death occurs. In fact, for myself, it started immediately after my Neurologist Dr McLeod gave me my grim diagnosis and prognosis that fateful day in March 2022.

Within minutes of my diagnosis and as soon as I left the hospital building, I called several people close to me and all were stunned, with most being emotional. What they were experiencing was anticipatory grief. One of the first people I called was my Go Global lead pastor and friend, Pete Anderson.

Pete prayed for me, and it was a prayer of hope, believing that God could heal me and, although he did not downplay the gravity of my diagnosis, it lifted my spirits. Having faith in God and trusting in Jesus was probably part of the reason why I remained quite calm, initially, after I was diagnosed and managed to drive the 60 miles home safely and without panic.

It is said that anticipatory grief will considerably affect the quality of life of a patient and the time he or she spends with his or her loved ones. But this does not need to be a negative. It can be a time for reconciliation or for strengthening relationships that are strained or distant. My relationship with my brother was strengthened when he came home from Aberdeen every weekend, and other family members rallied round me. The challenge for me and others with a terminal diagnosis is learning to focus on enjoying and valuing the life we have left, rather than focusing on the rigours and the prognosis of the condition we have.

There are two types of stigma that we suffer as a Christian, particularly a Church pastor. MND sufferers go from being reasonably fit to being dependent on carers in a relatively short space of time. For instance, as I write this chapter, I have gone from working full time only a year ago to needing showered, having a commode in my bathroom, using a rollator and being unable to cook. This can be quite demoralising, particularly if we have always been independent and self-sufficient.

To some, requiring constant assistance and needing a rollator and a wheelchair may be stigmatic, but I personally appreciate the help and assistance that I get and feel fortunate to be cared for with such love and empathy. Spiritual stigma, on the other hand, comes from the 'Health and Wealthers' or 'Name and Claimers', who believe that God heals everyone and if we are not healed that is down to a lack of faith or unrepentant sin. I am sure I am a disappointment to those with such beliefs as my story thus far of not being healed does not fit in with their theology.

I would imagine there are those who disregard their terminal diagnosis and live in denial. However, we are not called to live in denial. A good friend of mine who leads prayer ministry at Ellel Scotland told me that people with advanced cancer or other terminal illnesses have come there for prayer ministry and rest and those who denied having any illness in their body died within months.

Although there was a sense of surrealness after my diagnosis, I was fully aware of the enormity of the challenges ahead. In the first few months I did wake up some mornings absolutely pain free and feeling in spirit that I had been completely healed, only to stumble out of bed with the realisation that my legs were not as they once were and having to grapple to get support from the bedroom walls before keeling over.

I don't underestimate psychological impact of a terminal condition on a patient and his or her family. To watch the harrowing physical decline on anyone is heart-breaking, so it's understandable if some people may choose to deny that a loved one is critically ill.

Like Christ, we who follow Him must learn how to suffer without losing hope. We must learn to pray for our doctors, physicians, and scientists – not only that they might have the knowledge to help us, but also that they might have the courage to tell us when they cannot. Even more, we must understand that everyone handles a terminal diagnosis in their own way. Some people withdraw from public view and others are very public with their journey. And, finally, we must learn to sit with one another in the valley of the shadow of death while believing in the God of miracles.

As the reality of my mortality dawns on me more day by day and through many tears the simplest pleasures of this world have become sources of daily happiness and contentedness. It is only since I have become, for lack of a better term, more heavenly minded, that I can appreciate the blessings of everyday life for the astonishingly good divine gifts that they are.

I can sincerely say, without any sentimentality or super spirituality, that I am truly at peace. This is unusual for me because I have been a worrier all my life. I feel the power of prayer of many around the world who continue to pray for my healing and wellbeing.

I have never had so many days of sadness, but it is equally true that, although there are daily frustrations, I have never had more days filled with such comfort.

FEELING LOVED

Archbishop Desmond Tutu was diagnosed with cancer in 1997. As you would imagine, the diagnosis shook him to the core. He is quoted as saying: "I had no idea how much l was loved and cared for until l was diagnosed with cancer'". And l can honestly echo the late Archbishop's sentiments as l had no idea how much l was cared for and loved until l was diagnosed with this wretched MND – though l don't doubt that I still get under certain people's skin – but I am constantly reminded in Scripture of the importance of walking in love and grace.

Although painful in so many ways, living with a terminal illness offers us time to say "I love you" or "I deeply care about you" or to share our appreciation, and to make amends when necessary. When death occurs unexpectedly, we often regret not having had a chance to say and do these things.

During terminal illness, love is not only expressed through words, but also through inclusion and helping the ill person retain a sense of dignity. Even though a family member or close friend may be very ill and in need of care, they still value their privacy and self-worth. Personally, I am never left out of conversations I could be included in.

If you are living with someone terminally ill, don't speak about them as though they aren't there. Even if someone is critically ill and appears to be asleep or even unconscious, it's respectful and loving to leave the room to discuss their condition. They may still be able to hear you.

When we are changing or bathing, it is an expression of love to use a curtain or close the door to maintain our privacy. Always keep your patient covered with a towel when providing personal care. This is what I enjoy. Only one part of my body is uncovered at a time and it's never my private parts. Jennifer and my niece Zoe clearly want me looking as good as possible. They cut my finger and toe tails without me having to ask, and gently brush my hair. They also make sure I am shaven and smelling as good as possible.

Terminal illness can bring an almost sub-human to feel for the suffering person. The way that person had lived for so long has suddenly changed. Now they live with rollators, beeping machines, bedside monitors, lack of mobility, too-frequent visits from the Occupational Therapist, medical personnel coming and going, the weakening of their body, shortness of breath, and struggling to do what was once normal. The appetite has waned or disappeared, or eating becomes a messy affair.

What do we need in such a time? We need focus, touch, sensitivity, patience, and love. Unsightly things and unpleasant odours may be around, but that will not bother those who genuinely love and care with compassion.

When I was still a fairly new Christian, a pastor friend asked me to visit an elderly Christian man in a geriatric hospital in my hometown of Portsoy. He had no living family and didn't have many visitors. To be honest, the sights and odours were not the most pleasant to witness around his bed, but God gave me the compassion to stay, and to visit that lonely old man several times before he died. I had to get over my discomfort, realising how cold and callous it would be to deny a Godly man some much needed love and compassion before he was called home to glory.

All through my teens, twenties, and thirties I searched for love and happiness. But too often the kind of love I was looking for was influenced by lust and infatuation. I knew true love, joy and happiness were out there – I just had to find them. Like most people, I had spells of happiness but never for any length of time.

I remember being in primary school and thinking that if I had a new chopper bike, I would be happy. And at secondary school I reckoned when I left school and got a job, I would be happy. Then, after working as a painter for a few years, I felt that having my own business would make me happy.

Although it would be wrong to say I was unhappy, deep inside me there was still an emptiness and a feeling of discontent, there was still a lack of joy. Girlfriends and business success made me happy to a certain extent, but there was still a restlessness in my soul.

During these years of searching and striving I was oblivious to what true love really was. I did not understand the depth of 'Agape' love. Also called 'Agapi' in Hebrew and Greek, what the Bible says about love has a lot to do with the emotion of unconditional partiality, which is core to Christianity. It is to be shared with the broken, the marginalised, as well as the terminally ill.

Within Christianity, agape is the love originating from God or Christ for humankind. The biblical view of love is that it comes from God and is exhibited through us.

Biblical love is all-consuming, empowering, and lives in each of us. Our heart is the symbol of the love that resides in us, and God is the symbol of the love that reflects down on Earth.

THE COMPASSION, LOVE AND LEGACY OF FATHER DAMIEN

I had never heard of Father Damien until I was deeply moved by a blog on his life, example, and sacrifice by a dear Christian friend. Although the condition I battle daily is not contagious or stigmatic as the horrible disease he was eventually afflicted with, I am deeply challenged and mightily inspired by the story of Father Damien. During a casual google search I counted well over 30 books that had been written about his life and his legacy.

Father Damien was born Jozef ("Jef") De Veuster, in the village of Tremelo in rural Belgium on 3rd January 1840. From a young age, Jozef's dream was to be a priest. When he was old enough, He joined his older brother, Pamphile in the ministry. His superiors thought Jozef lacked sufficient education for the priesthood, however, but through hard work and his brother's help, he won their trust and confidence. After his theological studies, he went as a missionary to Hawaii and was ordained a priest in Honolulu in 1864.

In Hawaii he was deeply moved by the terrible condition of the lepers. From Scripture, as well as historical accounts, leprosy was considered a very ghastly disease. Lepers were detested. They were stoned and shunned. They were even killed.

As soon as a person showed the symptoms of leprosy, the authorities sent them to Molokai, where they were cut off from the rest of the world. Being exiled to Molokai was regarded as a death sentence by the Hawaiians. This place may have looked like a glimpse of heaven, but to many who lived there it was hell on earth.

Father Damien found that once the sufferers were sent to the island nothing was done for them. Healthy people refused to work there for fear of catching the disease. With no proper water supply or housing, the 600 lepers were left to nurse each other.

In 1873, answering the call for volunteers on the island, Father Damien, arrived at the isolated leprosy settlement of Kalaupapa. At his arrival, he spoke to the assembled lepers as "one who will be a father to you, and who loves you so much that he does not hesitate to become one of you; to live and die with you". At first repulsed by the smell of rotting flesh, he learns to dress ulcers and goes on to help build 300 buildings for the leprosy patients on Molokai.

During this time, Father Damien cared for the lepers and established leaders within the community to improve the dire standard of living. Father Damien aided the colony by teaching, painting houses, organising farms, and the construction of chapels, roads, hospitals, orphanages, and churches. He also dressed residents, dug graves, built coffins, ate food by hand with them and lived with the lepers as their equal.

Father Damien passed up many opportunities to leave Molokai. So great was his love and compassion for those he served that he wrote to his brother saying: "People pity me and think me unfortunate, but I think of myself as the happiest of missionaries". Father Damien's sacrifice was an embodiment of Christ's: "No one has greater love than this, to lay down one's life for one's friends". (John 15:13) For 16 years, Father Damien worked in Hawaii, providing love and comfort to the lepers of Molokai.

In December 1884, while he was preparing to bathe, Father Damien inadvertently put his foot into scalding water, causing his skin to blister. He felt nothing and realised that he had contracted leprosy after working in the colony for 11 years. This was the standard way for people to discover that they had been infected with leprosy. Despite his grim diagnosis, Father Damien worked even harder.

With an arm in a sling, a foot in bandages, and with his leg dragging, Father Damien knew that his death was near. He was bedridden on 23 March 1889, and died of leprosy at 8:00 a.m. on 15 April 1889, at the age of 49.

A fierce critic of Father Damien, The Reverend Doctor Charles Hyde wrote of the Belgian born priest soon after his death: "The simple truth is, Father Damien was a coarse, dirty man, headstrong, and bigoted".

He also suggested that, among other scathing criticisms, his contracting leprosy was a result of yielding to a vice which may have rung true or untrue. If they were true, then praise God that despite our flaws and imperfections He can still use us mightily until we draw our last breath. And that sinlessness is only the divine attribute of Jesus Christ Himself.

Father Damien may have been confined to a slow, rotting, stigmatised death, but what he offered the other lepers, who were condemned to a slow death, was the truth that Christ is Lord, and that God is love. He became a leper among the lepers; he became a leper for the cause of the lepers. He suffered and died alongside them, stooping to the lowest of the low, as his Lord and Saviour did, knowing that he would rise again in Christ.

ONE DAY AT A TIME

After receiving my MND diagnosis in March 2023, I naturally prayed for physical healing. I also prayed that I would not only be able to deal with having the condition, but also that I may be able to rejoice in the tough journey ahead. I prayed for more trust in this part of God's plan for me. Since then, I have seen God use these trials to build my faith. I firmly believe He desired to show the power of the gospel in my daily life, and that through my condition somehow His name may receive glory and honour.

To feel fear is still a consistent temptation. My condition has no recognised medical remission as it devours muscles all over my body. Now that I have reached the landmark of 60, God's veiled purpose behind all the uncertainty is hard to deal with at times. No wonder Paul writes: "We were so utterly burdened beyond our strength . . . to make us rely not on ourselves but on God who raises the dead". (2 Corinthians 1:8–9)

Because of my condition I now constantly cry out to the Lord for mercy. I literally cannot rely on my own strength to survive. If we hope to escape the constant despair and debilitating fear that often comes with medical incurable disease – or whatever unique fears we may face – we must rely on the Lord to carry us through and strengthen us, one day at a time. It is utterly masochistic not to do so.

One thing I must maintain is a sincere attitude of gratitude for all I have to be thankful for. To face each day with gratitude and appreciation, however much I am struggling physically.

Author Amy Weatherly wrote: 'Some people could be given an entire field of roses and only see the thorns in it. Others could be given a single weed and only see the wildflower in it'. Perception is a key component to gratitude and gratitude a key component to joy. Or in the words of Robert Louis Stevenson: "Life is not a matter of holding good cards, but of playing a poor hand well". We have no control over the cards we are dealt in life, but we can control how we deal with our hand.

"Do not worry about tomorrow, for tomorrow will worry about itself. Each day has enough trouble of its own". (Matthew 6:34)

I've spent far too much of my life worrying, even as a Church pastor. Here's how it worked: My mind would conjure up a number of possible scenarios, mainly all negative, of course. I figured out how to respond to each one: "If this happens, then …" And at some subconscious level, I convinced myself that if I imagine and prepare for enough scenarios, I won't be surprised by whatever comes my way.

But I have learned to meditate on the words of the apostle Paul in – 2 Corinthians 4:16-17 – "So we do not lose heart. Though our outer self is wasting away, our inner self is being renewed day by day. For this light momentary affliction is preparing for us an eternal weight of glory beyond all comparison".

There are almost 160 000 poor souls worldwide who never woke up this morning. Many were elderly or terminally ill and although they will still be mourned, their passing was probably not a surprise. But many of this number died young or suddenly in seemingly good health, leaving their devastated families in a state of shock.

I like what Charles Kingsley the 19th century Church of England minister wrote: "Do today's duty, fight today's temptation and do not weaken and distract yourself by looking forward to the things we cannot see, and could not understand if you saw them".

Life is like the oil within a lamp. It can be measured, but the pace at which it burns depends on how the dial is turned day by day, how bright and fierce the flame. And there is no predicting whether the lamp might be knocked to the ground and shatter when it could have shone brightly for a good while longer. Such is the unpredictability and fragility of life. And as long as our lamp burns, we have life, and we have purpose.

A daily Devotional I read posed the question how we would we react if our bank credited our account by the sum of £86,400 every day; on the condition that the money was completely spent the same day. If not, it's withdrawn from our account. The process is then repeated the next day and every other day with £86,400 being credited to our account daily. I'm sure most of us would have no hesitation in using the money every day! Similarly, God blesses us with 86,400 seconds of life every day, which can never be reclaimed if not used! Let us therefore use the time wisely.

Taking a day at a time is almost a worn-out cliché but it is so true and simply profound. It's not about ignoring or sugar-coating the harsh realities we may well be facing, but rather a sobering check for our often anxious and restless souls. Only in the last year have I truly learned to appreciate the value of taking one day at a time.

Looking back and yearning for the 'normal' past can push us to an endless pit of melancholy, while looking too far ahead might be filled with many empty promises, leaving us in despair. Although, at the same time we take for granted the importance and blessing of the people who add value to our lives, and the small, seemingly insignificant things we do today.

A successful US country songwriter by the name of Marijohn

Wilkin drifted away from her faith after finding success. At a time of crisis and personal desperation, she stopped at a church for some counselling and prayer. The young minister who was on duty had apparently asked her during the conversation whether she had ever considered being thankful to God for her problems. She went home and pondered that statement, then began to play her piano and the words of a song came to her.

Needing some help to complete the lyrics that she had written down, she approached Kris Kristofferson who helped her with some of the remaining words. You have likely heard the song.

The completed song goes like this:

I'm only human, I'm just a woman
Help me believe in what I could be, and all that I am
Show me the stairway, I have to climb
Lord for my sake, teach me to take, one day at a time.
One day at a time sweet Jesus, that's all I'm asking from you
Help me believe in what I could be, and all that I am
Show me the stairway, I have to climb
Lord for my sake, teach me to take, one day at a time.
One day at a time sweet Jesus, that's all I'm asking from you

Ultimately, MND may take my independence, but I won't let it break my spirit.

EPILOGUE

PITY ME NOT

(EULOGY INSPIRED BY JOZANNE MOSS)

Pity me not:
For I am the rich one
With treasures stored up in the sky.

Pity me not:
God's Spirit's inside me
I don't feel alone or afraid.

Pity me not:
Though my body is limp
My spirit sours up there on high.

Pity me not:
Though my life may seem shortened
Today is all we can count on.

Epilogue: Pity Me Not

Pity me not:
My life may seem useless
But my Father chose me for His glory.

Pity me not:
My joy is complete,
For my purpose before me is clear.

So, pity me not
No, pity me not
I'm right where God wants me to be.
Pity me not:
For our time in this life
Withers and wastes away.

It's the life after this
When we stand with the Son
That will last for eternity.

So, pity me not:
No, pity me not
I'm right where God wants me to be.